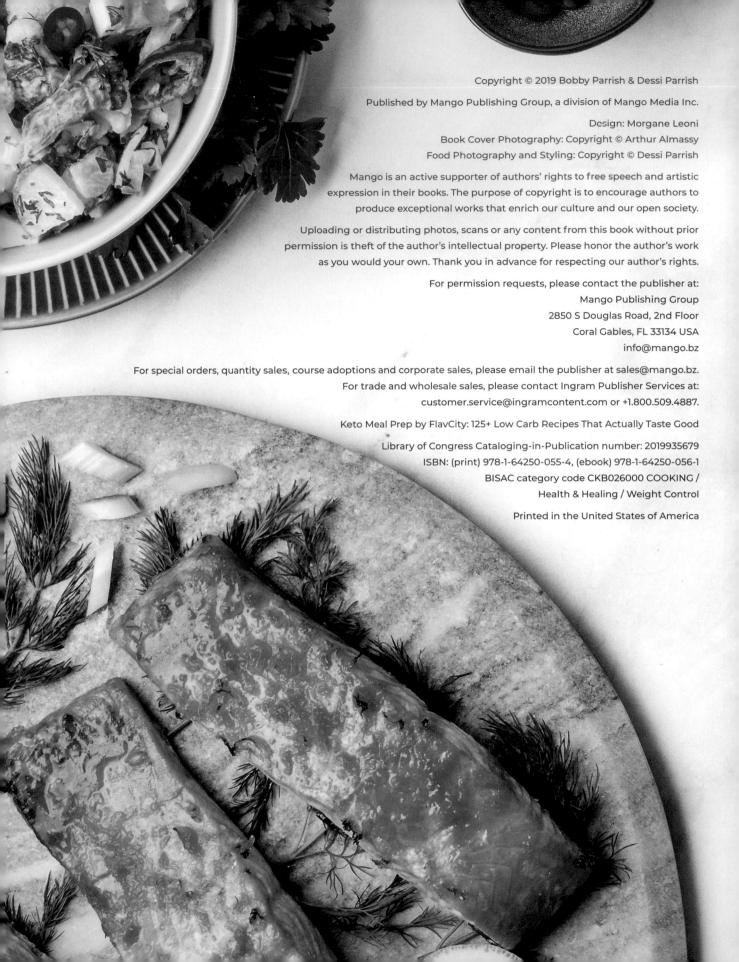

For permission requests, please contact the publisher at:
Mango Publishing Group
2850 S Douglas Road, 2nd Floor
Coral Gables, FL 33134 USA
info@mango.bz

For special orders, quantity sales, course adoptions and corporate sales, please email the publisher at sales@mango.bz.
For trade and wholesale sales, please contact Ingram Publisher Services at:
customer.service@ingramcontent.com or +1.800.509.4887.

Keto Meal Prep by FlavCity: 125+ Low Carb Recipes That Actually Taste Good

Library of Congress Cataloging-in-Publication number: 2019935679
ISBN: (print) 978-1-64250-055-4, (ebook) 978-1-64250-056-1
BISAC category code CKB026000 COOKING /
Health & Healing / Weight Control

Printed in the United States of America

Keto Meal Prep

by

flavcity

125+ Low Carb Recipes That Actually Taste Good

BOBBY PARRISH & DESSI PARRISH

Mango Publishing

Coral Gables

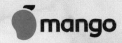

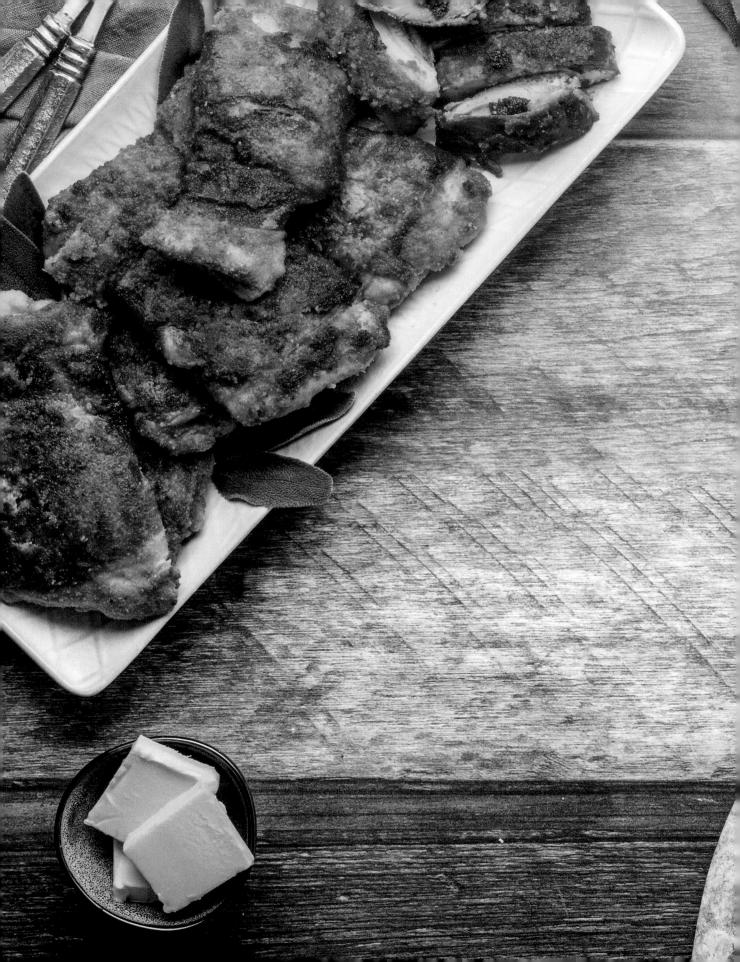

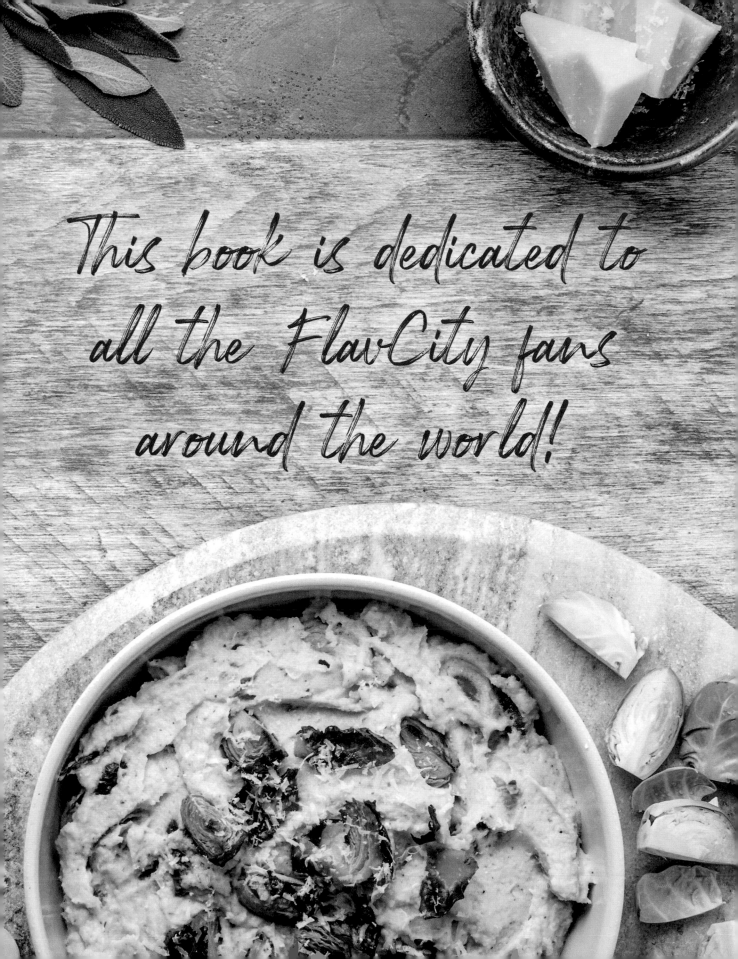

This book is dedicated to all the FlavCity fans around the world!

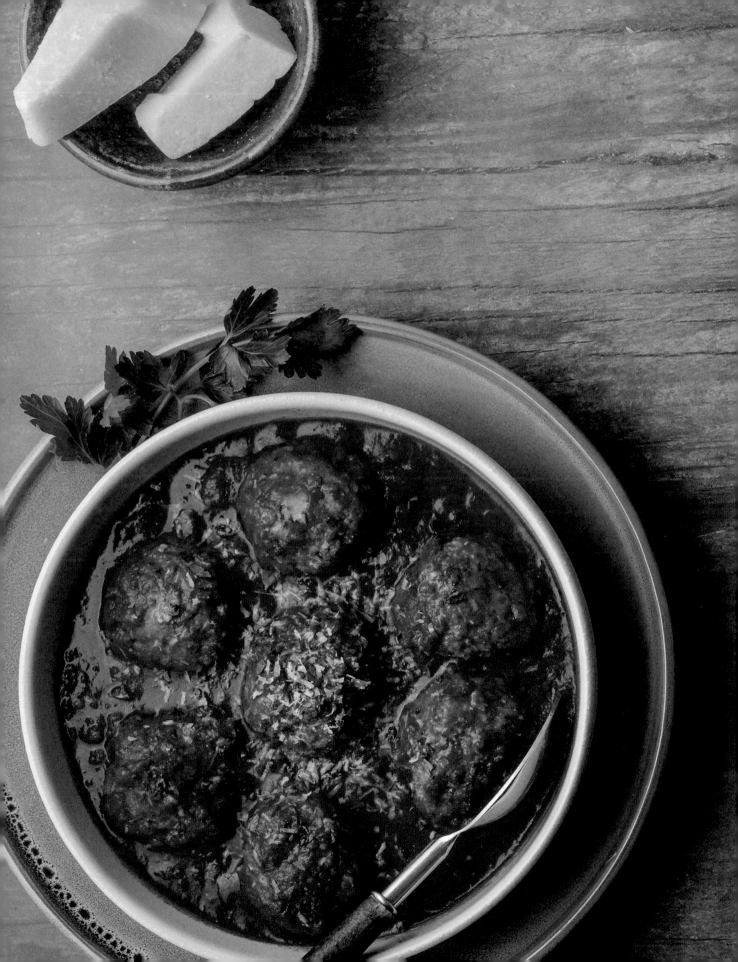

CONTENTS

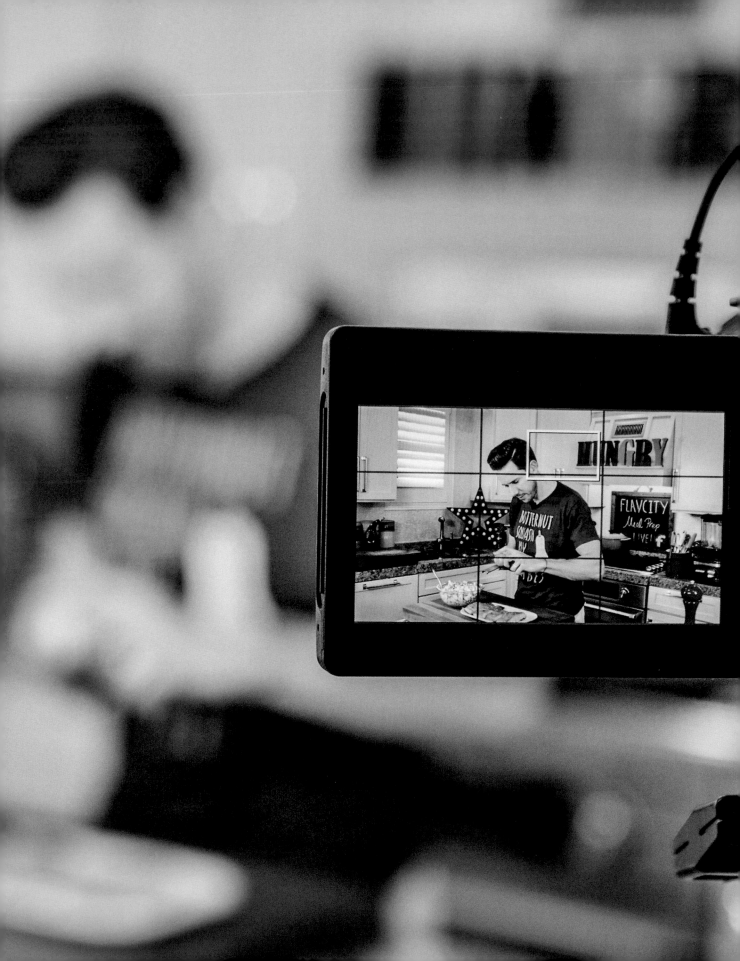

INTRODUCTION

Raise your hand if you're tired of eating boring healthy food. That's what I thought, which is why my mission from day one of starting the FlavCity YouTube channel was to make healthy food sexy, exciting to make, and so darn tasty! I can make you one promise: there's not one recipe in this cookbook that won't slap your taste buds silly with flavor. Nope, I did not throw in the towel and put a couple of lazy-butt recipes in this book. I would never do that to my flavor family.

This cookbook has 50 low-carb keto meal prep recipes that taste good—actually epic—and 25 individual keto recipes. Keep in mind that each meal prep has 2 to 3 components, so there are well over 125 recipes in this book that you can mix and match for endlessly tasty keto combinations.

Having a social media following of over one million family members—that's what I like to call you guys—has really helped me understand the food you crave and the recipes you want to eat. I don't make videos on the FlavCity YouTube channel just to see my perfectly quaffed hair. I make them to motivate our viewers to get into the kitchen and make healthy, homemade recipes that taste great and help you achieve your dietary goals. Keep in mind that Dessi does my hair; you don't want to see what it looks like if I try to do it!

I went to one of the most prestigious culinary schools in the country—my mom's kitchen. Have you heard of it? Perhaps you are a graduate too? Mom sparked the culinary bug in me when I was a little shorty, and I have never looked back. From cooking in my tiny little college apartment, to hosting dinner parties for my friends when I graduated, all I ever wanted was to be in the kitchen creating recipes. That's why after working in finance (as an options trader) for more than ten years, I had to quit my job and go all in with cooking. We had this incredible YouTube channel, social media accounts, and blog that were growing, and I wanted to put all of my efforts into that. Dessi quit her job in 2018, and amazing things started happening. We had a number of viral videos (check my grocery store haul videos), built a new blog, and finally got motivated to write a keto cookbook after so many fans requested it.

It's funny to think that all of this started because I got rejected from *Food Network Star*. I wanted to be on that show so badly because I knew I would win and get my own show. So, when they gave me the cold shoulder, I decided to start a YouTube channel, and I think things have turned out pretty well. We publish one or two cooking videos every weekend on the FlavCity YouTube channel, daily videos and posts on Instagram with nightly IG stories of what I'm making for dinner, and recipe videos on the FlavCity Facebook page. And don't forget about our shiny new blog that is the home to every recipe and video ever made. It looks so good because Dessi has a computer science MS degree and can pretty much do anything. She's amazing like that. As if that was not enough, you get the bonus of watching my dad come over most nights for dinner on the FlavCity IG stories. He pretty much has a cult following and is known for his no-nonsense reviews of my recipes.

Every recipe in this book has detailed macros and nutrition information which are a pain to calculate, so I hope you appreciate it! Almost every recipe has a video tutorial on YouTube, and, if you ever have a question, just shoot me an email or a DM on Instagram. I actually reply to almost all messages even though it makes my eyes burn from staring at the screen for so long. You guys are totally worth it! Enjoy these keto meal prep recipes, as I truly believe they are some of the best ones out there, and welcome to the FlavCity family! #KeepOnCooking

PS: Make sure to tag me on social media using #FLAVCITY when you make the recipes from this book. I love seeing your creations!

QUICK REFERENCE ICONS:

	Meal Prep (indicates this recipe is suited for a meal prep)
	No Eggs (indicates recipes contains no eggs)
	No Dairy (indicates recipes contains no dairy)
	No Nuts (indicates recipes contains no nuts)
WHOLE30	Indicates recipe is Whole30 diet compliant
PALEO	Indicates recipe is Paleo diet compliant
Tip	Insight on a particular recipe from the authors
You Tube	Video Tutorial (indicates there's a video tutorial on YouTube for this recipe)
★★★★★	Comments by real FlavCity fans on Social Media and Blog

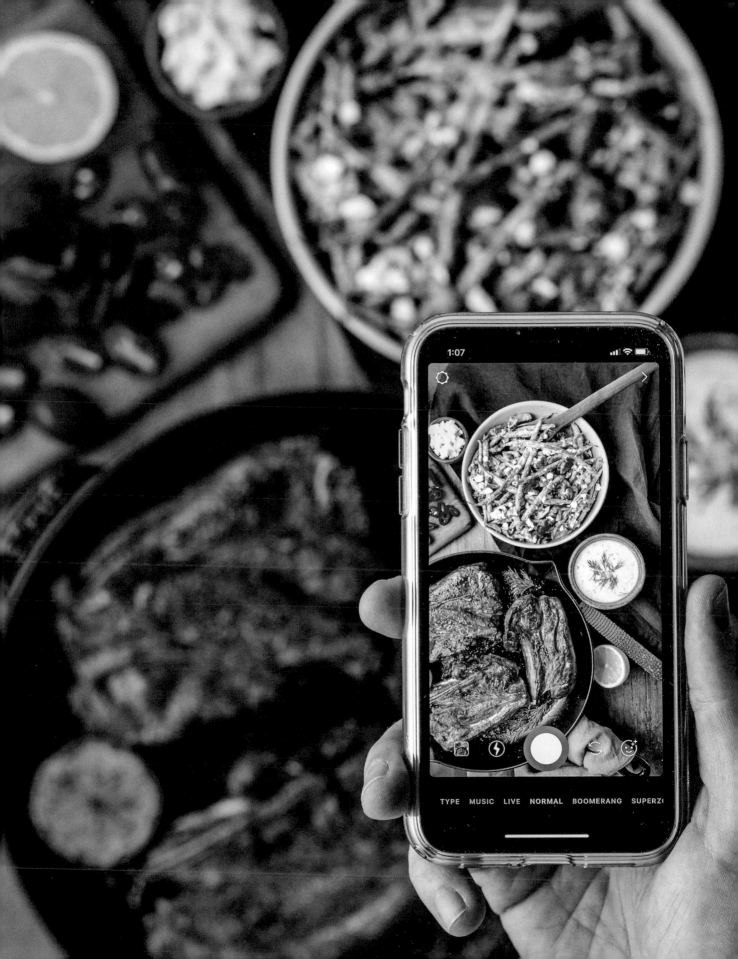

TIPS TO MEAL PREP LIKE A BOSS

Here are some rock-solid tips to help you meal prep for the week like a boss. I'm not talking about lame ideas like making a shopping list, so don't stress out. These are actionable ideas that will help with your meal prep lifestyle.

Kitchen Tools to Help You Meal Prep like an Iron Chef

A chef is only as good as his tools, and these are my must-have tools to navigate the kitchen and rock your meal prep recipes like a boss. All of these kitchen tools can be found on **www.flavcity.com/shop**.

LARGE CAST-IRON PAN:

If it was good enough for grandma, it's good enough for you. You can cook everything except for eggs in your cast-iron pan. Nothing distributes heat quite like it, and nothing sears meat the way cast iron does.

LARGE NON-STICK PAN:

Do you see where I am going? Bigger is better! You can always add fewer ingredients to a pan, but you can't increase its surface area. You are going to need a non-stick pan to cook seafood, veggies, and anything you don't feel like busting out your cast-iron pan for.

CUTTING BOARDS:

You will need two cutting boards for all of that meal prep you are going to do—a wooden cutting board and a plastic one (for raw proteins). A large wooden board will handle everything except raw meat and protein which have bacteria that can breed in the wood and cause contamination. A large surface area will prevent you from chasing veggies on the floor—trust me, I've been there. A plastic cutting board should have rubber around the edges, so it does not slide around when being used to prep for recipes.

EIGHT-INCH CHEF'S KNIFE:

99 percent of the chopping you will do for meal prep can be done with a good chef's knife. I have ones that cost fifteen dollars and ones that cost over two hundred dollars. You can choose either one and don't need to bother buying any other knife besides a paring knife.

MICROPLANE ZESTER:

Fans of the FlavCity YouTube channel do not call me "obsessed with zest," or #ObZest, for no reason. I love how you can zest fresh lemon, orange, or lime over the top of any dish and totally transform the flavor and add a subtle pop of acid. The microplane is also my favorite way to grate Parmesan and Pecorino Romano cheese as it creates this snow shower that is so darn beautiful.

LEMON AND LIME JUICER:

Once you have zested the citrus, you are likely going to squeeze some juice into something. Instead of using your hands and feeling the burn on that fresh paper cut, you can use a citrus juicer that can squeeze way more juice out than your hands can. Trust me.

HALF-SHEET TRAY:

People always ask me how my sheet trays stay so clean. It's because I buy new ones as soon as the old ones get nasty. They are cheap, durable, and a meal prep essential for all of the veggies and chicken you will be cooking in the oven.

SPLATTER GUARD:

Sometimes the cleanup process takes more time than the actual cooking! Make sure that never happens again by using a guard to cover the pan while you are cooking; it blocks the oil from going all over the place.

PROBE THERMOMETER:

Never overcook another piece of chicken or meat by using a digital probe thermometer; this gadget stays inside the meat while it's baking in the oven. It has an alarm that tells you when it has reached the desired cooking temperature.

What's in Your Pantry?

Having a stocked pantry is the key to adding flavor and creating various types of meal prep recipes at a moment's notice. When you have a fully loaded pantry, you can literally make any meal you want, and these items will last you a long time.

Make sure you have a variety of **spices** on hand. My favorites are smoked paprika, cumin, ancho chili powder, turmeric, and coriander. Try to buy spices from a spice shop or the bulk section of Whole Foods. The ones at the grocery store have been sitting on the shelves for gosh knows how long, and ground spices start to lose their flavor after three months.

Make sure to always cook with kosher **salt** and finish with Maldon or flakey sea salt, if desired. Keep on hand different **vinegars** like balsamic, red wine, and rice wine vinegar. Cooking and finishing **oils** are a must. Carry olive oil, avocado oil, and expeller pressed grape seed oil for cooking with heat and use extra virgin olive oil to drizzle over a finished dish.

Carry **condiments** in your pantry like tamari soy sauce or coconut aminos, toasted sesame oil (store in fridge), hot sauce, liquid stevia, and coconut milk.

Costco Is Your Best Friend

This may seem obvious, but stock up on non-perishable items at Costco like nut butters, nuts, almond flour, coconut milk, and cooking oils. You will be using lots of those items to meal prep, so why not save some money? Watch my Costco grocery haul video on YouTube for more inspiration and lots of mean comments.

Why I Love Glass Meal Prep Containers

Glass meal prep containers are much safer than plastic ones and perfect for warming in the oven or microwave. I don't care what they say about plastic meal prep containers being safe for the microwave—that is total garbage—the chemicals from plastic are not safe for the food: end of story.

FAQ

Here are some questions going through your head now, because I know you guys so well!

HOW LONG CAN I STORE MEAL PREP?

Each recipe in this book has storage instructions, but most meal prep recipes can be stored in the fridge for five days or frozen for two to three months. Make sure to keep sauces and dressings separate from protein and salads, and only dress them right before you want to enjoy them. Some meal prep items like cauliflower rice and salads don't freeze well and get soggy when defrosted.

WHAT IS THE BEST WAY TO REHEAT MEAL PREP?

Each recipe in the book has reheating instructions, but the best way to reheat meal prep is in a 350°F oven for 7—10 minutes. If using the microwave, place a wet paper towel over the container and make sure not to overheat, as the food can dry out. You can also use the HotLogic Mini—it's a great way to reheat meals at work or school.

HOW DO I CALCULATE MACROS?

Luckily you have me, and I did all of the hard work for this book! In case you want to calculate your own macros for a different recipe, there are four trusted websites I use. You need to check multiple sites because I often find errors on some.

- www.fatsecret.com
- www.eatthismuch.com
- www.nutritionix.com
- www.myfitnesspal.com

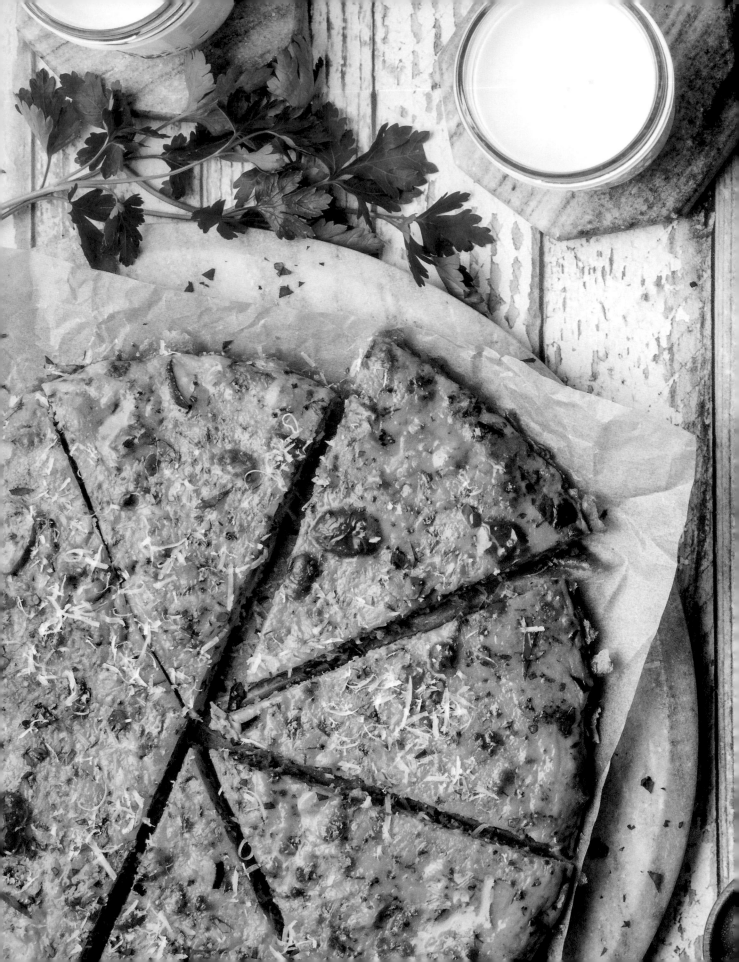

WAKEY WAKEY, EGGS AND BAKEY!

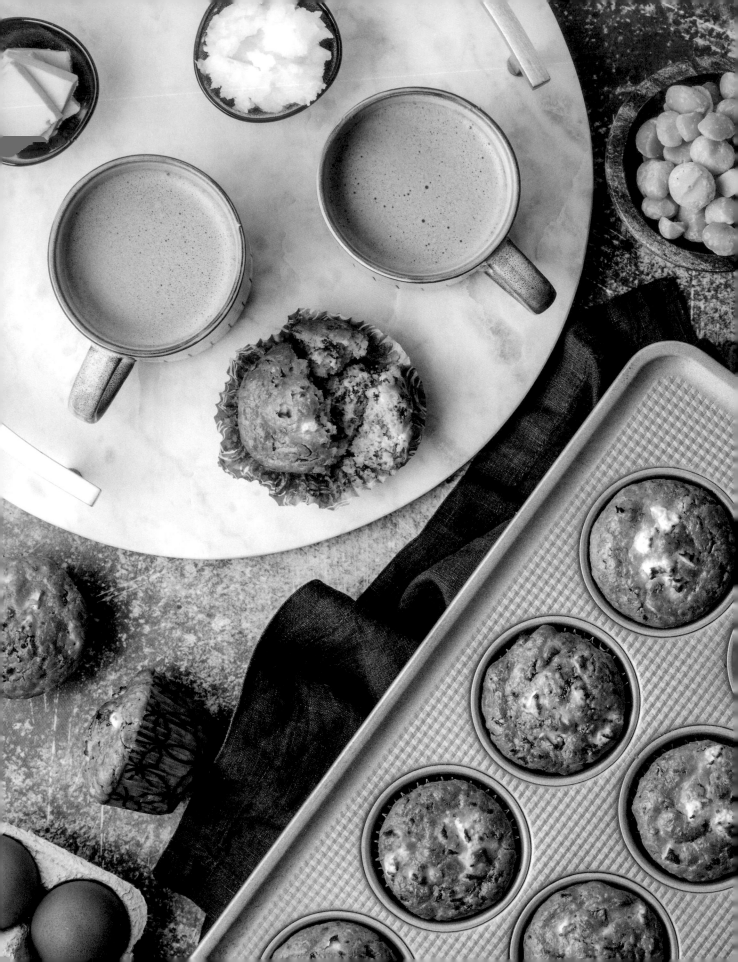

PREP TIME: **10 MINUTES** • COOKING TIME: **25 MINUTES** • MAKES: **9 MUFFINS**

SPINACH AND FETA MUFFINS
WITH BUTTER COFFEE

Dessi is kind of a genius when it comes to baking; for me, it's my archenemy. You may notice this is the same batter used to make the fat bread and bagels, except this time it's loaded with spinach and salty feta and served with the elixir from the gods known as butter coffee.

Tip Yes, I know macadamia nuts are expensive, but you really need them for this recipe. You can substitute the coconut butter with runny almond butter if desired.

You Tube To watch the video tutorial for this recipe, search "FlavCity keto muffins" and "FlavCity butter coffee" on YouTube.

FOR THE MUFFINS:

- 1 cup macadamia nuts, unsalted and roasted if desired
- 5 eggs
- ¾ cup coconut butter, mixed well
- ½ teaspoon kosher salt
- 1 teaspoon baking soda
- Zest of ½ lemon
- 1 tablespoon fresh lemon juice
- 1 cup feta cheese, crumbled
- 1 cup frozen & chopped spinach, thawed
- 3 tablespoons grated Parmesan cheese

FOR THE COFFEE:

- 1 cup of hot coffee
- ½ tablespoon organic virgin coconut oil
- ½ tablespoon unsalted grass-fed butter

Make the muffins: Preheat the oven to 350°F and make sure the oven rack is set in the middle. Add the macadamia nuts to a food processor or a powerful blender, and process for about 30 seconds until almost creamy. While the machine is running, add the eggs one at a time, making sure each one has been incorporated into the batter before adding the next one. Turn the machine off and add the coconut butter and salt, and process until smooth and creamy. While the machine is off, add the baking soda and lemon zest and juice, and process for 10–15 seconds.

Transfer the batter to a large bowl and add the feta cheese. Next, you must squeeze out as much liquid from the thawed spinach as possible. Otherwise, it will mess up the consistency of the muffins. Once that is done, add it to the batter and mix well. Spray a muffin tin with non-stick spray or rub them with avocado oil or butter. Fill the muffin tins just about all the way up and top with grated Parmesan. Bake in the oven for 25 minutes. The muffins are ready when a toothpick is inserted and comes out clean and they are nicely golden brown. Remove from the oven and allow to cool for 10 minutes before removing and serving. Enjoy!

For the butter coffee, blend hot coffee with coconut oil and butter on high for 30 seconds. Make sure to securely hold a kitchen towel over the top of the blender.

STORAGE AND REHEATING: Store muffins in the fridge for three days or freeze for two months. Thaw frozen muffins and warm in a 300°F oven for 3–5 minutes.

MACROS

per muffin (makes 9):
319 calories
3.22 grams of net carbs
7.42 grams of total carbs
28.7 grams of fat
4 grams of fiber
8.6 grams of protein

MACROS

for the coffee:
122 calories
0 carbs
14 grams of fat
0.4 grams of protein
0 fiber

★★★★★

"Delicious muffins!! These have become instant staples for me! Flavor is spot on; the texture and nutrition are perfect. Thank you for the recipe!" —**Michael J.**

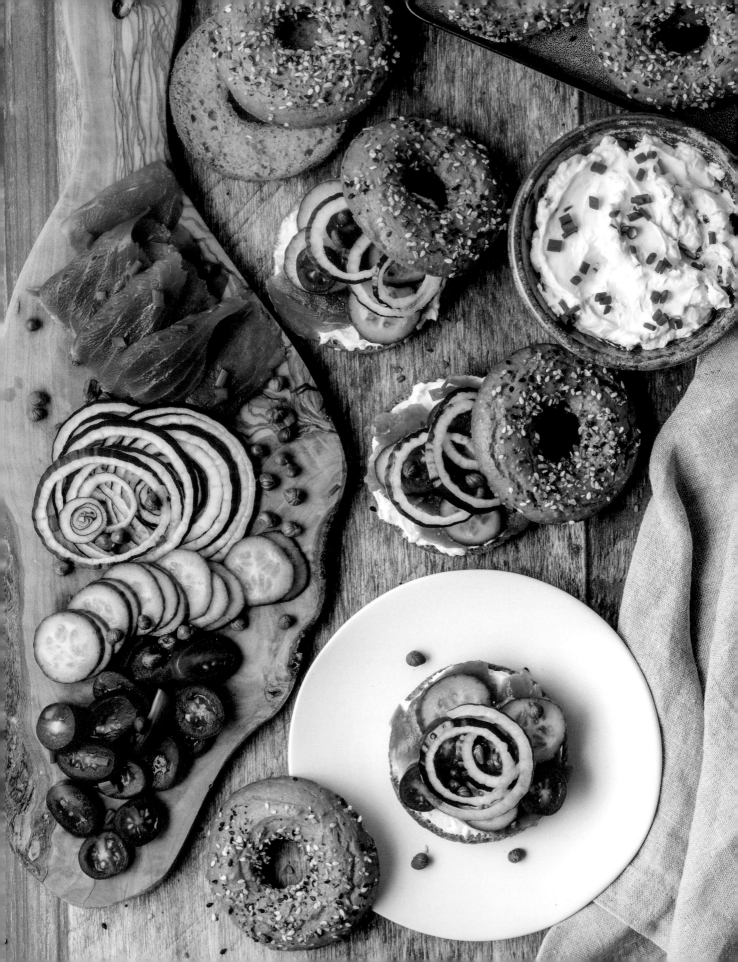

PREP TIME: **15 MINUTES** • COOKING TIME: **20 MINUTES** • MAKES: **10 BAGELS**

PALEO

DESSI'S
EVERYTHING BAGELS

Weekend mornings just have not been the same since you cut out bagels on the keto diet, right? Well, now you can make an epic bagel, cream cheese, and smoked salmon sandwich again, thanks to these tasty and oh-so-cute bagels from Dessi! Ok, they are not chewy and doughy like real bagels, but it's the best you are gonna get on keto, my friends.

You Tube | To watch a video tutorial for this recipe, search "FlavCity keto bagels" on YouTube.

INGREDIENTS:

- 1 cup macadamia nuts, unsalted and roasted if desired
- 5 eggs
- 1 cup coconut butter
- ½ teaspoon kosher salt
- 1 teaspoon baking soda
- Zest of ½ lemon
- 1 tablespoon fresh lemon juice
- 1–2 tablespoons everything bagel seasoning

Preheat your oven to 350°F and make sure the oven rack is set in the middle. Add the macadamia nuts to a food processor or a powerful blender and process for about 30 seconds, until almost creamy. While the machine is running, add the eggs one at a time, making sure each one has been incorporated into the batter before adding the next one. Turn the machine off and add the coconut butter and salt, and process until smooth and creamy. Next, while the machine is off, add the baking soda and lemon zest and juice, and process for 10–15 seconds.

Spray some non-stick cooking spray in a bagel or donut pan. Add the batter to a large zip-top bag, cut off one of the corners, and pipe the batter into the tin. Tap it on the counter a couple times. Sprinkle as much of the everything bagel seasoning as you would like, and use your finger to gently press it down into the batter so it does not fall off. Bake in the oven for about 22 minutes or until nicely golden brown on top. Remove from the oven, allow to sit in the tin for 5 minutes, and then transfer to a cooling rack for 15 minutes.

Slice the bagels and enjoy!

STORAGE AND REHEATING: Bagels will keep for three days in the fridge in an airtight container or can be frozen for three months.

MACROS

per bagel (makes 10):
283 calories
2.5 grams of net carbs
6.6 grams of total carbs
26.1 grams of fat
4 grams of fiber
5.4 grams of protein

★★★★★

"These bagels just made my breakfast. Eggs, bacon, bagel, cream cheese!! Yaasss honey! These taste even better the next day!" —**Robyn R.**

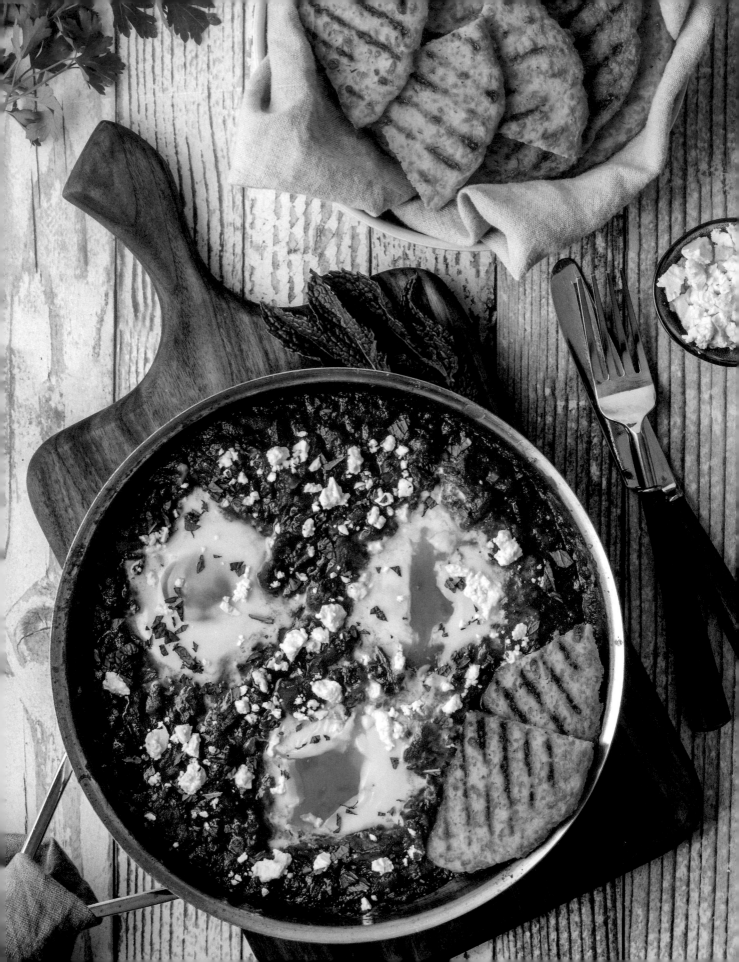

PREP TIME: **10 MINUTES** • COOKING TIME: **25 MINUTES** • MAKES: **2 MEALS**

SHAKSHUKA
WITH FETA AND MINT

I started noticing many restaurants serving shakshuka and said to myself, "Hey, I can make that at home for much cheaper and way better." Turns out I was right! It's a North African one-pan tomato and egg dish that is perfect for a lazy Sunday morning. You can't mess it up.

Tip | When a recipe calls for canned tomatoes, make sure to only buy Italian San Marzano canned tomatoes. They are grown in the rich volcanic ash from Mount Vesuvius and have the best flavor.

You Tube | To watch a similar video tutorial for this recipe, search "FlavCity shakshuka" on YouTube.

INGREDIENTS:

- 1 green bell pepper, sliced
- ½ cup red onions, diced
- 4 cloves garlic, minced
- ¼ cup roasted assorted bell peppers
- 1 teaspoon smoked paprika
- 1 teaspoon cumin
- ½ teaspoon cayenne pepper
- 20 ounces of canned tomatoes, chopped
- 4 eggs
- ¼ cup feta cheese, crumbled
- Fresh mint, minced
- Parsley, minced
- Kosher salt and fresh pepper
- Olive oil

Preheat a twelve-inch skillet over medium heat along with 1 tablespoon of oil. Add the green peppers, onions, ¼ teaspoon salt, and a few cracks of pepper. Cook for 12 minutes or until the veggies are soft, stirring often. Add the garlic and cook for 3 minutes. Add the roasted peppers, paprika, cumin, and cayenne pepper and cook for 1 minute. Add the chopped canned tomatoes with juice along with ½ teaspoon of salt and a few cracks of pepper. Bring to a simmer and cook until the tomatoes have reduced and the sauce is somewhat thick, about 15–20 minutes. Turn the heat to medium-low. Then use a spoon to make indentations for the eggs, and crack the eggs directly into the spots. Season the tops of the eggs with a pinch of salt and pepper, cover with a lid or sheet pan, and cook for 7–10 minutes or until the egg whites are set.

Remove from the heat, garnish with the feta cheese and herbs, and enjoy! You can use the keto pita bread recipe from page 165 to dip into the tomato sauce. You can even char the pita bread in a hot grill pan to make it crusty.

STORAGE AND REHEATING: You can store the shakshuka in the fridge for three days and reheat in the oven.

MACROS | **for the entire pan of shakshuka:**
682 calories
28 grams of net carbs
44.8 grams of total carbs
42.5 grams of fat
36 grams of protein
16.75 grams of fiber

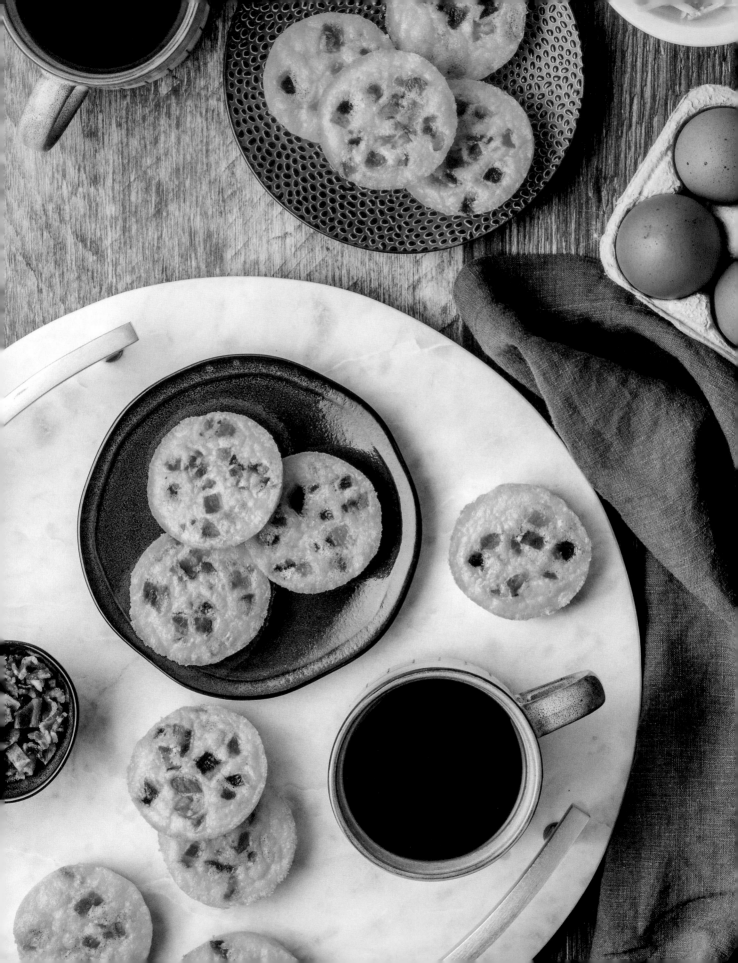

PREP TIME: **5 MINUTES** • COOKING TIME: **30 MINUTES** • MAKES: **10 EGG BITES**

COFFEE SHOP EGG BITES

I really like the sous vide egg bites from Starbucks, but I hate paying $4.75 for an order of two. So, I decided to make a homemade keto version that not only tastes better, but also only costs $1.27 for two. As you can tell by the fan comments, people were very pleased!

 Tip | This recipe works best with a silicone muffin pan. The egg bites just slide right out, which doesn't always happen with the metal muffin tins.

 | To watch the video tutorial for this recipe, search "FlavCity egg bites" on YouTube.

INGREDIENTS:

- 10 eggs
- 1 cup of shredded Gruyère or Swiss cheese
- ½ cup full-fat cottage cheese
- ½ teaspoon kosher salt
- Couple cracks of fresh black pepper
- 4 slices of cooked paleo (sugar-free) bacon

First, make sure to cook the slices of bacon before making the egg bites. Next, preheat the oven to 300°F and place a baking dish that is filled with 1 inch of water on the bottom rack. This will create a humid environment and help the eggs cook evenly. Add the eggs, cheese, cottage cheese, salt, and pepper to a blender and blend on high for 20 seconds until light and frothy. Spray a regular-size muffin tin with non-stick spray and fill each cup ¾ the way to the top with the egg mixture. Divide the chopped bacon equally among the muffin tins and bake in the oven for 30 minutes or until the center of the egg bites are just set. Remove from the oven and let cool for 5 minutes; then use a spatula or fork to carefully remove them from the muffin tin. Enjoy!

STORAGE AND REHEATING: Store the egg bites in the fridge for three days or freeze for two to three months. Reheat in a microwave or warm oven.

MACROS

per egg bite (makes 10):
144 calories
1 gram of net and total carbs
10.4 grams of fat
13.5 grams of protein
0 fiber

★★★★★

"I LOVE these!!! They are absolutely delicious and REALLY easy to make. Perfect for taking to work for lunch. My new fav!!! Thanks, Bobby!!!" —**Kristina P.**

"Heaven in my mouth! I love the Starbucks version but can't justify the price. Love making these in bulk and freezing! On point! Thanks for making it easy!" —**Damaris**

"I don't know what really goes inside there, so that's why I google searched and found you. Now, we both can enjoy these goodies at home, and I think I will switch the bacon for veggies and, voila, baby has her yummy breakfast. Great job!!!! THANK YOU!" —**Luka**

"Awesome recipe. They're an instant favorite for a quick breakfast on the go. They taste just like the Starbucks egg bites, but I feel so much better knowing exactly what is in them. Thanks for doing the hard work and figuring this recipe out." —**C. Mitchell**

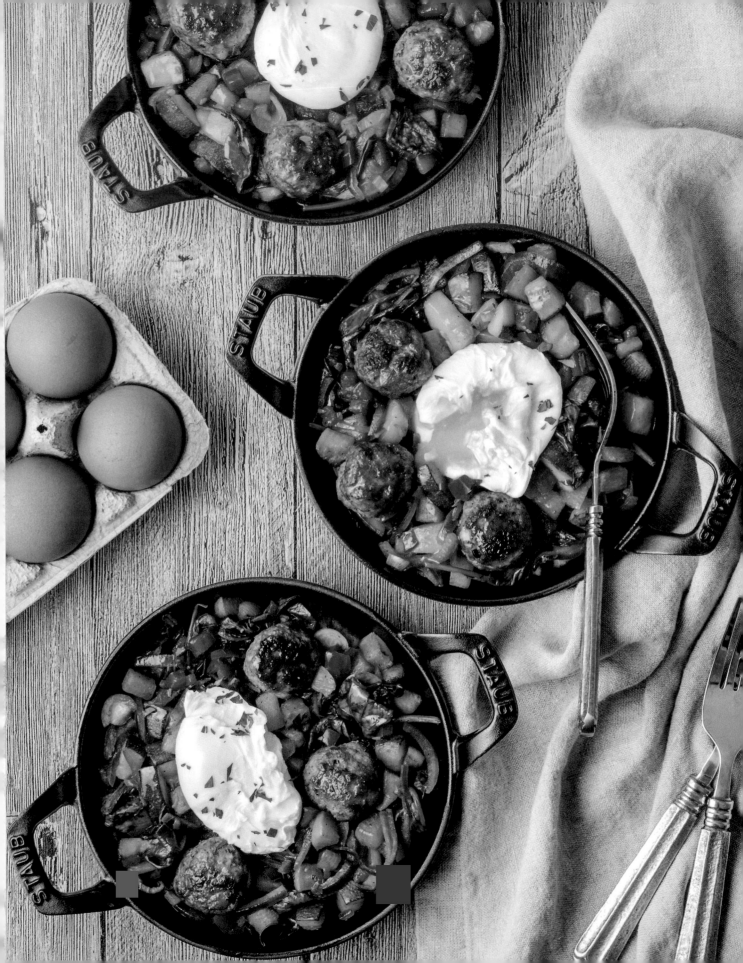

PREP TIME: **15 MINUTES** • COOKING TIME: **20 MINUTES** • MAKES: **3 MEALS**   PALEO / WHOLE30

MINI MEATBALL
BREAKFAST HASH

I refuse to go out for brunch! I don't have the patience or stamina to wait an hour for a table when my tummy is rumbling. I need to feed the machine. Plus, most places have starchy potatoes and low-quality eggs. This keto and paleo hash is truly one of a kind. And who doesn't want to eat meatballs for breakfast!?

To watch a similar video tutorial for this recipe, search "FlavCity breakfast hash" on YouTube.

INGREDIENTS:

- 8 ounces of ground lamb or any ground meat
- ¾ teaspoon smoked paprika
- ¾ teaspoon cumin
- ½ teaspoon dried oregano
- ¼ teaspoon cayenne pepper
- 1 teaspoon vinegar, any flavor
- 3 eggs
- 3 turnips (12 oz), peeled and diced
- 1½ large zucchini, diced
- 1 green bell pepper, diced
- ½ red onion, thinly sliced
- 6 ounces baby spinach
- Olive or avocado oil
- Kosher salt and fresh pepper

MACROS

per serving of hash (makes 3):
378 calories
12.2 grams of net carbs
17.5 grams of total carbs
27.3 grams of fat
22.9 grams of protein
5.2 grams of fiber

Make the mini meatballs: Add the ground lamb to a medium-sized bowl and season with the smoked paprika, cumin, oregano, cayenne, ½ teaspoon salt, a few cracks of pepper, and mix until just combined using your hands. Form mini meatballs by dipping your hands in cold water and rolling them (this will prevent the mixture from sticking to your hands). Make sure they are small, or they won't cook through.

To poach the eggs, bring at least 6 inches of water to a bare simmer in a pot and add 1 teaspoon of any flavor vinegar. Cracks the eggs (one at a time) into a mesh strainer and let the water from the whites drain away. Place the eggs in ramekins; then make a vortex in the water using a spoon, and carefully tip in the first egg. Repeat with remaining eggs and cook for exactly 3 minutes. If the shape gets kind of funky, just use a spoon to help the egg whites form properly around the yolk. This is important right after they go in the water. Remove eggs, dip in cold water for 5 seconds, and set aside.

For the hash, preheat a large pan just over medium heat for 2 minutes with 2 teaspoons of oil. This works best with a cast-iron pan but non-stick also works. Add the meatballs and cook until crusty on all sides and cooked through—about 8 minutes. Remove meatballs, add a shot of oil to the pan if needed, and add the turnips to the pan. Cook for 5 minutes or until they become slightly crusty. Add the zucchini and cook for 3 minutes. Next, add the bell pepper. The goal is to cook the veggies in order of what takes the longest. Once the veggies have nice color and have softened a bit, add the red onion along with ½ teaspoon of salt and a few cracks of pepper. Cook for 3 minutes. Next, add the spinach, and cook until wilted. You may have to add the spinach in 2–3 batches and allow it to wilt down before adding more. Check for seasoning as you may need more salt. Remove from heat, add the meatballs back, serve with the poached eggs, and enjoy!

STORAGE AND REHEATING: Everything will keep in the fridge for three days. You can reheat the poached eggs in warm water for 30 seconds or until the yolk is soft. Reheat the meatballs and hash in a hot pan or in the microwave. This meal prep cannot be frozen.

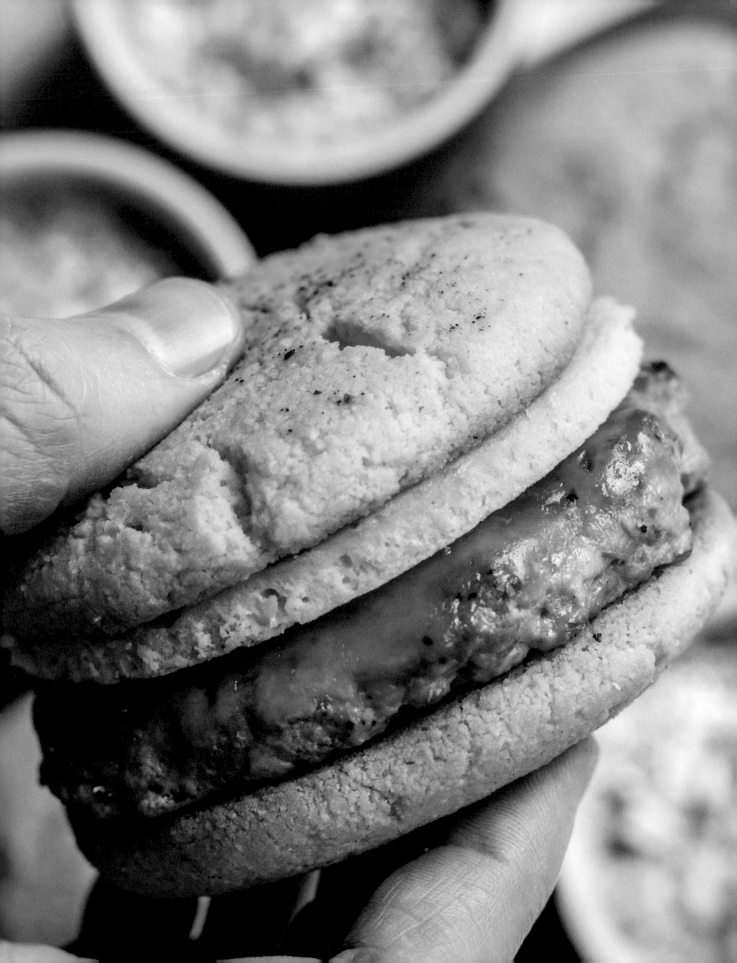

PREP TIME: **25 MINUTES** • COOKING TIME: **45 MINUTES** • MAKES: **5 MEALS**

BREAKFAST SANDWICH
AND COCONUT CHIA SEED PUDDING

Breakfast meal prep recipes are one of the most popular requests on our YouTube channel, and it's safe to say they don't have these brekkie sandwiches on the menu at Micky Ds! The almond flour biscuits make the perfect low-carb bun and the chia seed pudding is so easy to make; I'm loving it.

FOR THE CHIA PUDDING:

- 1 cup unsweetened almond milk
- 1 cup full-fat coconut milk
- 1 teaspoon no sugar vanilla extract
- ½ teaspoon ground cinnamon
- Tiny pinch of salt
- Stevia drops to taste
- ¼ cup plus 2 tablespoons chia seeds

| FOR THE BISCUITS:

- 2 cups almond flour
- 2 teaspoons baking powder
- ½ teaspoon garlic powder
- ½ teaspoon onion powder
- 2 eggs, beaten
- ½ cup melted butter
- Kosher salt and fresh pepper

FOR THE SANDWICH:

- 5 eggs
- 3 chicken sausage links, about 3.5 ounces each
- ¼ cup grated sharp cheddar cheese
- 2 ice cubes
- Avocado oil
- Kosher salt and fresh pepper

Tip | Cooked eggs will only last for three days in the fridge, which is why the sandwich portion of this recipe makes three servings. You may want to double it and keep some in the freezer or make more eggs later in the week.

Tip | For best results, allow the chia seed pudding to rest overnight in the fridge so it can really set up.

  To watch the video tutorial for this recipe, search "FlavCity sausage breakfast sandwich" on YouTube.

Make the chia pudding by combining everything but the chia seeds and stevia in a bowl and whisking well. Taste the liquid and add enough stevia drops to taste. Add the chia seeds, a little at a time, and whisk very well. Let the pudding sit 10 minutes and then whisk it very well. Repeat this process one more time then move the pudding to the fridge to set up overnight. The next day it will be thick and have the consistency of pudding. Pudding can stay in the fridge for five to seven days.

For the biscuits, preheat oven to 350°F. In a large bowl, sift in 2 cups of almond flour. If you don't have a sifter, make sure there are no large clumps of flour. Add baking powder, ½ teaspoon salt, some pepper, onion and garlic powder, and mix well. In a small bowl, whisk the eggs and add the melted butter and mix well. Pour the wet batter over the dry batter and use a spatula to mix well.

Line a sheet tray with parchment paper or tin foil and fill a ¼ cup measuring cup about 80 percent full of dough. Use your hands to form the biscuit to 2.5 inches in diameter and place on the sheet tray. You want all the biscuits to be the same size; they will spread out a bit while baking. Crack a little black pepper over the top of the biscuits and bake for 15–16 minutes or until golden brown. Remove and let cool completely. This recipe makes 8 biscuits.

To make the eggs that go on top of the sandwich, preheat oven to 400°F. Crack 5 eggs in a large bowl and whisk vigorously for 30 seconds until light and airy. Add ¼ teaspoon of kosher salt and a couple cracks of pepper, and whisk a few more times. Preheat an eight- or nine-inch non-stick pan over medium heat with 1 teaspoon of oil and add the eggs. Use a spatula to continuously stir the eggs, and, once they start to set a little, transfer the pan to the oven and bake for 7–8 minutes. Remove from oven and use a spatula to transfer the entire egg disk to a plate or cutting surface. Use a drinking glass or ring mold to cut out circles that roughly match the size of the biscuits. Set aside.

Make the sausage patties: Cut the chicken sausages out of their casings and form them into patties slightly wider than the biscuit. To make uniform patties, I like to cover a large mayo or peanut butter lid with plastic wrap and push the sausage down into the mold. Then pull the plastic wrap and meat out of the lid and finish forming the patty. Preheat a pan (preferably cast-iron) just below medium-high heat for 2 minutes with 2 teaspoons of oil. Add the patties and cook for 3–4 minutes on the first side, or until a nice brown crust forms, and then flip and lower the heat to medium. Add an equal amount of cheese on top of each patty, place 2 ice cubes in the pan, and immediately put a lid on the pan or cover it with a sheet tray. The ice will help the cheese melt evenly. Cook another 3 minutes and then remove the chicken patties from the pan.

Assemble the sandwich by placing a sausage patty and an egg disk on a biscuit. Use another biscuit for the top bun. Enjoy!

STORAGE AND REHEATING: The chia seed pudding will last for five to seven days in the fridge but can't be frozen. Keep the biscuits in an airtight container in the fridge. The sausage patties will last for five days in the fridge; the eggs will only last for three days. Both can be frozen for two to three months. Reheat the sausage patty in a 350°F oven for roughly 10 minutes or place a wet paper towel over a container and reheat in microwave.

MACROS	per chia pudding (makes 5 servings):	MACROS	per sausage, cheese, egg combo (makes 3):	MACROS	per biscuit (makes 8):
	168 calories		265 calories		259 calories
	2.2 grams of net carbs		1.1 gram of net carbs		2 net grams of carbs
	7.3 grams of total carbs		1.5 grams of total carbs		4.2 grams of total carbs
	13.8 grams of fat		16.8 grams of fat		25.8 grams of fat
	4.25 grams of protein		27.1 grams of protein		6 grams of protein
	5.1 grams of fiber		0 fiber		2.25 grams of fiber

★★★★★

"I can go on and on about this recipe. It was so good. I made it this morning before work. Even though I used my grounded chicken breast, it came out delicious. I followed every step on YouTube. Thanks so much. I love you and your wife's videos..." —**Joy**

"This breakfast was OMG amazing! Even my non-keto family loved it. I love your recipes, tips, and humor. Thanks for helping me stay keto strong." —**JJZ**

"Soooooo this breakfast biscuit just saved my life! Thank you because it's been so hard to get my boyfriend to commit to keto, but he actually loves the way almond flour tastes! We even made slightly bigger biscuits and made little prep pizzas. They freeze well too. Thank you, thank you, thank you!" —**Breona**

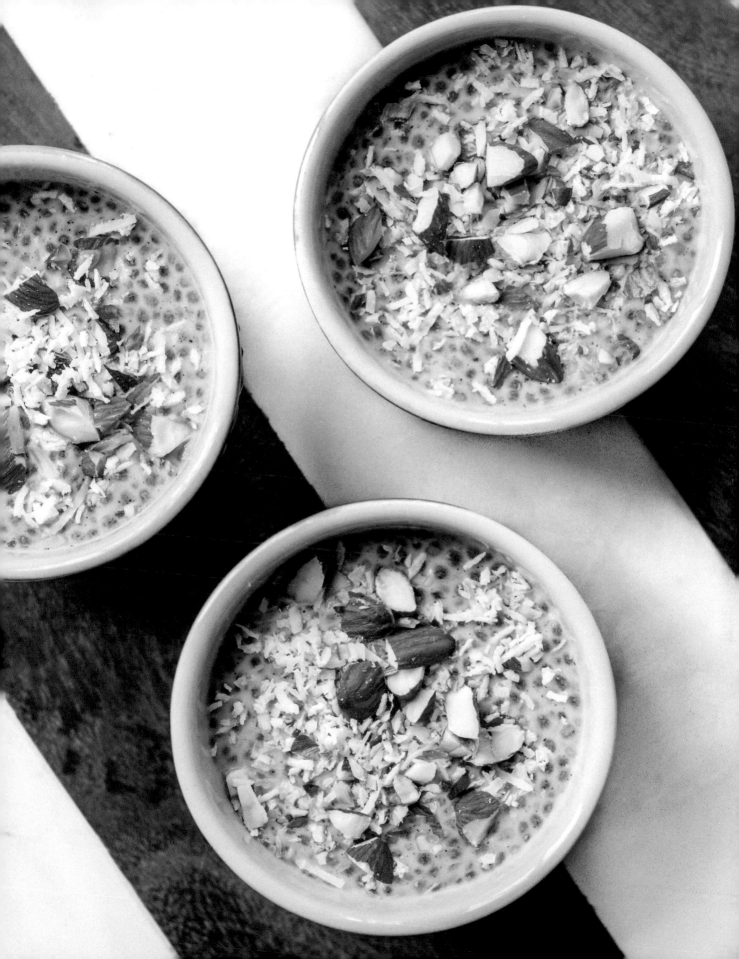

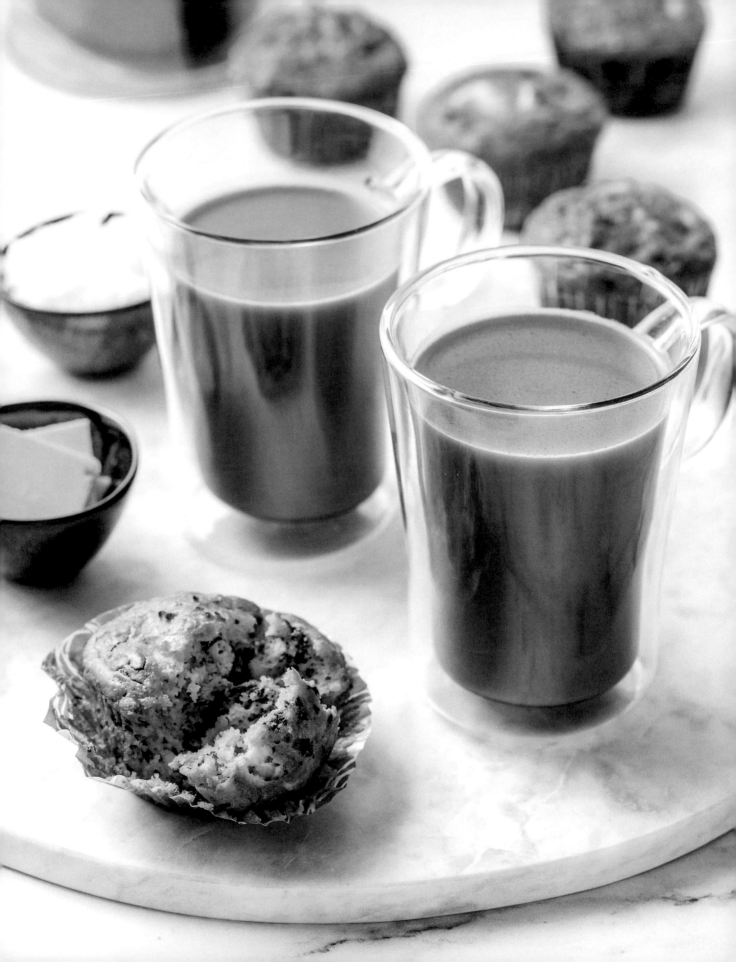

PREP TIME: **5 MINUTES** • COOKING TIME: **1 MINUTE** • MAKES: **1 CUP OF COFFEE**

MOCHA BUTTER COFFEE

You know those days when you're feeling naughty and want one of those six-dollar Starbucks drinks to satisfy the craving? Make this instead. It's cheaper and is actually good for you, unlike those drinks that are actually a dessert in a cup.

 To watch the video tutorial for this recipe, search "FlavCity butter coffee" on YouTube.

INGREDIENTS:

- 1 cup of hot coffee
- ½ tablespoon organic virgin coconut oil
- ½ tablespoon grass-fed unsalted butter
- 2 teaspoons cocoa powder, sugar free
- 4–5 drops liquid stevia
- 1–2 tablespoons coconut cream or heavy cream
- ¼ teaspoon cinnamon

Blend everything together on high for 30 seconds and make sure to securely cover the top of the blender with a kitchen towel in case the coffee spills out. Enjoy!

Muffins: This coffee goes great with our spinach and feta muffins, see recipe on page 19.

MACROS

per cup of coffee:
169 calories
1.8 grams of net carbs
3 grams of total carbs
19 grams of fat
1.3 grams of protein
1.2 grams of fiber

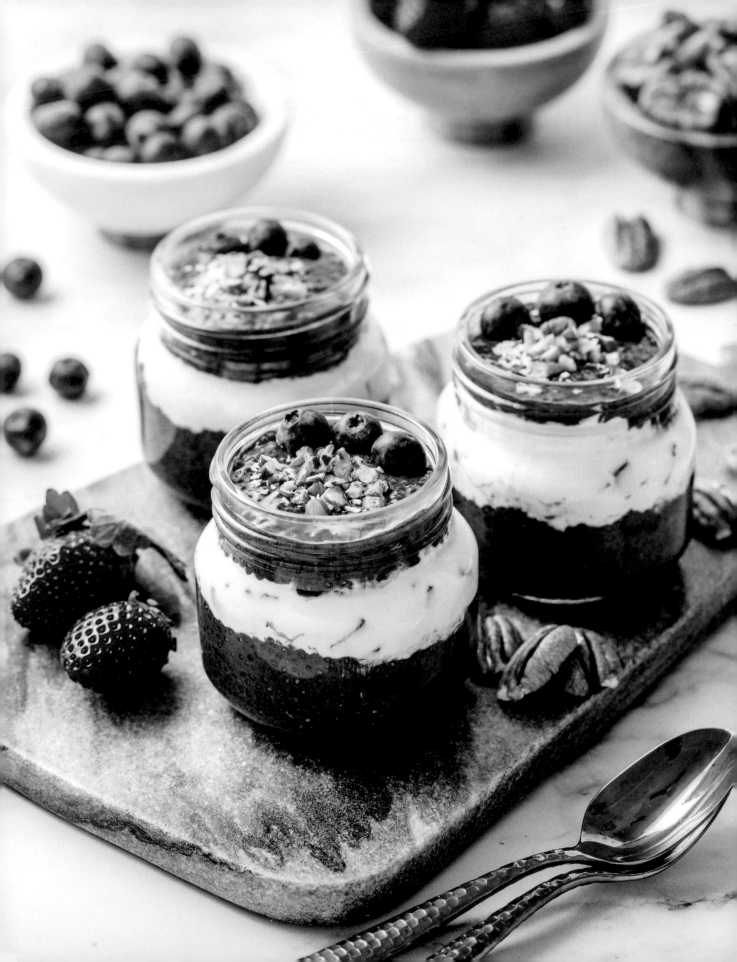

PREP TIME: **5 MINUTES** • ACTIVE COOKING TIME: **5 MINUTES** • MAKES: **5 SERVINGS**

PALEO

CHOCOLATE CHIA SEED PUDDING

I could eat this creamy chia seed pudding every day and never get tired of it! Feel free to change up the flavors and toppings as desired.

 Tip

Make sure the chia seeds are whisked very well before putting in the fridge to set up overnight. If the seeds stick to each other, they won't thicken the pudding properly.

 You Tube

To watch the video tutorial for this recipe, search "FlavCity chocolate chia seed" on YouTube.

INGREDIENTS:

- 1 cup unsweetened almond milk
- 1 cup full-fat coconut milk
- 2 tablespoons unsweetened cocoa powder
- 1 teaspoon cinnamon
- 1 teaspoon no sugar vanilla extract
- Tiny pinch of salt
- Stevia drops to taste
- ¼ cup plus 2 tablespoons chia seeds

Make the chia pudding by combining everything but the chia seeds and stevia in a bowl and whisking well. You can also blend on very low speed in a blender. Taste the liquid and add enough stevia drops to taste. Add the chia seeds—a little at a time—and whisk very well. Let the pudding sit 10 minutes and then whisk it very well again. Repeat this process one more time and then move the pudding to the fridge to set up overnight. The next day it will be thick and have the consistency of pudding. Feel free to add whole Greek yogurt or keto fruit like blueberries and raspberries.

STORAGE AND REHEATING: Pudding can stay in the fridge for five to seven days.

MACROS

per serving (makes 5):
173 calories
2.65 grams of net carbs
8.5 grams of total carbs
14.1 grams of fat
4.7 grams of protein
5.8 grams of fiber

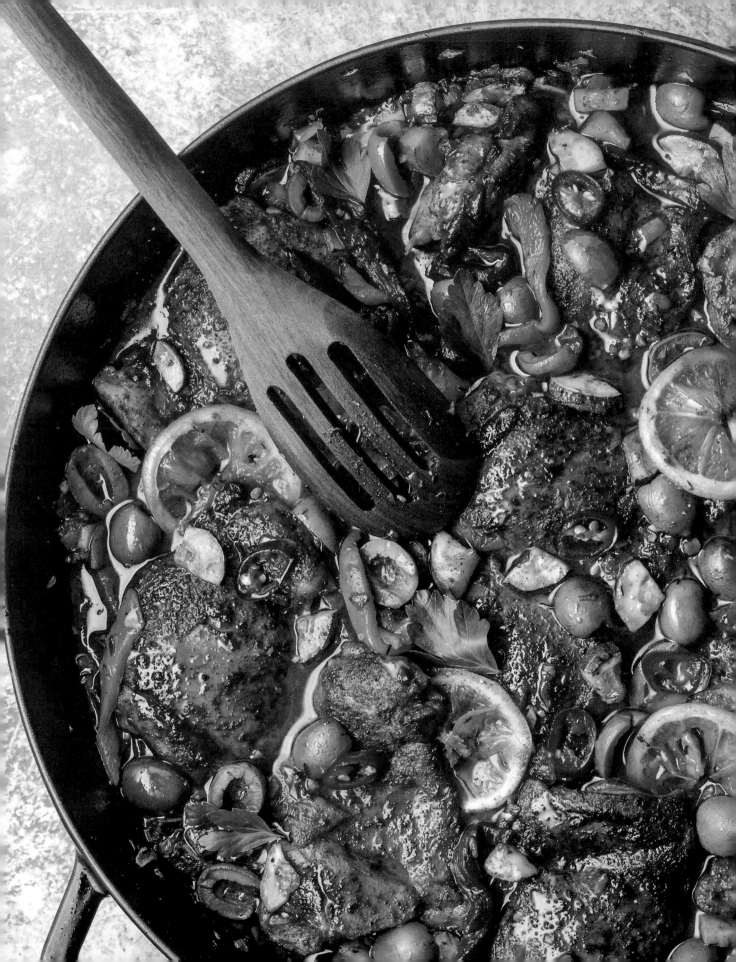

WINNER, WINNER, CHICKEN DINNER!

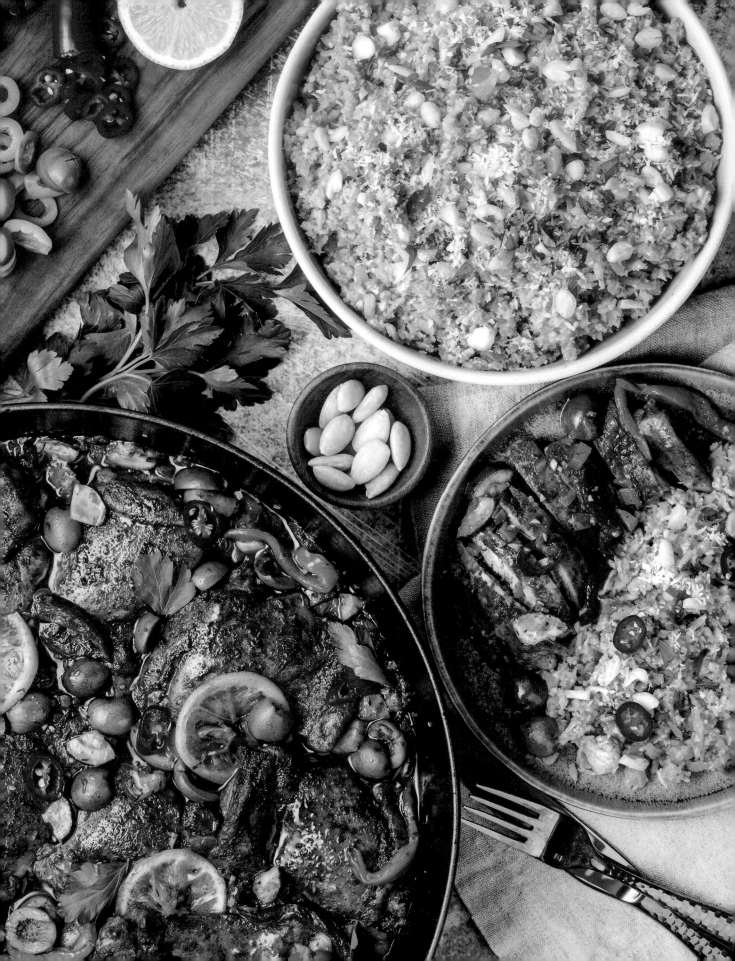

PREP TIME: **20 MINUTES** • COOKING TIME: **40 MINUTES** • MAKES: **5 MEALS**

PALEO / WHOLE30

MOROCCAN CHICKEN STEW
WITH GOLDEN CAULIFLOWER RICE

Choosing my favorite recipe would be like having to choose a favorite child, but I am going on the record and saying this is my favorite recipe in the book! This one-pot chicken stew is full of flavor and the golden cauliflower rice with turmeric and coconut milk will make you forget about starchy white rice.

 Tip | Yes, I know there are a lot of ingredients listed in this recipe, but feel free to skip a few. It won't ruin the recipe if you don't have roasted peppers, red chilies, or an orange for zesting. Recipes are guides, not written in stone (unless you're baking, then you better follow the rules)!

 You Tube | To watch the video tutorial for this recipe, search "FlavCity Moroccan Chicken" on YouTube.

FOR THE CHICKEN:

- 1 teaspoon smoked paprika
- 1 teaspoon cumin
- ½ teaspoon ground coriander
- ¼ teaspoon ground cinnamon
- ⅛ teaspoon ground cloves
- 10 boneless and skinless chicken thighs
- ½ onion, chopped
- 1 medium zucchini, cubed
- ½ teaspoon dried thyme
- 3 cloves garlic, minced
- 6 ounces jarred roasted peppers, sliced
- ½ cup good quality green olives, pitted and halved
- 1½ cups chicken stock/broth
- 4 thin slices of lemon
- ½ red chili, thinly sliced, or pinch of red pepper flakes
- 1 teaspoon parsley, chopped
- Avocado or olive oil
- Kosher salt and fresh pepper

FOR CAULIFLOWER RICE:

- 1 large head of cauliflower
- ½ onion, chopped
- 3 cloves garlic, minced
- 1 teaspoon fresh grated ginger
- 1 tablespoon ground turmeric powder
- 1 cup full-fat coconut milk
- 3 tablespoons unsweetened shredded coconut flakes
- ¼ cup blanched almonds or walnuts, chopped and roasted if desired
- Zest of ½ lime
- Zest of ½ orange
- 1 tablespoon parsley, chopped
- ½ red chili, thinly sliced
- Avocado oil
- Kosher salt and fresh pepper

For the chicken, make the spice rub by combining the smoked paprika, cumin, coriander, cinnamon, and cloves in a small bowl, and mix well. Season the chicken with a generous pinch of salt and half the spice rub on one side, flip and repeat. Preheat a wide pan just under high heat for 2 minutes. Add 1 tablespoon of oil, wait 30 seconds, and add the chicken to the pan. If your pan is not big enough to fit all the chicken, do this in two batches. Cook the chicken for 2–3 minutes (or until the crust is golden brown and crusty), flip and repeat, and remove from pan. Lower the heat to medium, add 2 teaspoons of oil to the pan and add the onions, zucchini, thyme, ¼ teaspoon salt and a few cracks of pepper. Cook for 10 minutes, stirring often. Add the garlic and cook for 3 minutes. Then add the roasted peppers, olives, and chicken, along with any juices and enough chicken stock to come halfway up the side of the chicken. Tuck the lemon slices around the chicken and add the sliced chilies. Bring the liquid to a boil, reduce to a simmer, and cook uncovered for 20–25 minutes, or until the stock has reduced considerably and can be used as a sauce. Move the chicken around the pan a couple times so everything cooks evenly. Sprinkle parsley over the dish when the chicken is ready and set aside.

STORAGE AND REHEATING: Everything will keep in the fridge for five days or can be frozen for two to three months. Reheat in a 350°F oven for 7–10 minutes. If using the microwave, cover the container with a wet paper towel and make sure not to overheat—otherwise the chicken will get dry.

MACROS

per chicken breast (makes 5):
285 calories
0 carbs
11.5 grams of fat
51 grams of protein
0 fiber

MACROS

per serving of spinach (makes 5):
381 calories
7.8 grams of net carbs
13.1 grams of total carbs
31 grams of fat
12.5 grams of protein
4.8 grams of fiber

★★★★★

"I made this a week after the video came out, and it was really fantastic! The chicken was easy to cut, so smooth and delicious! The spinach: I don't think I've ever had so much flavor in my spinach before... I highly recommend this recipe, and I will for sure cook it again and again." —**Pascal**

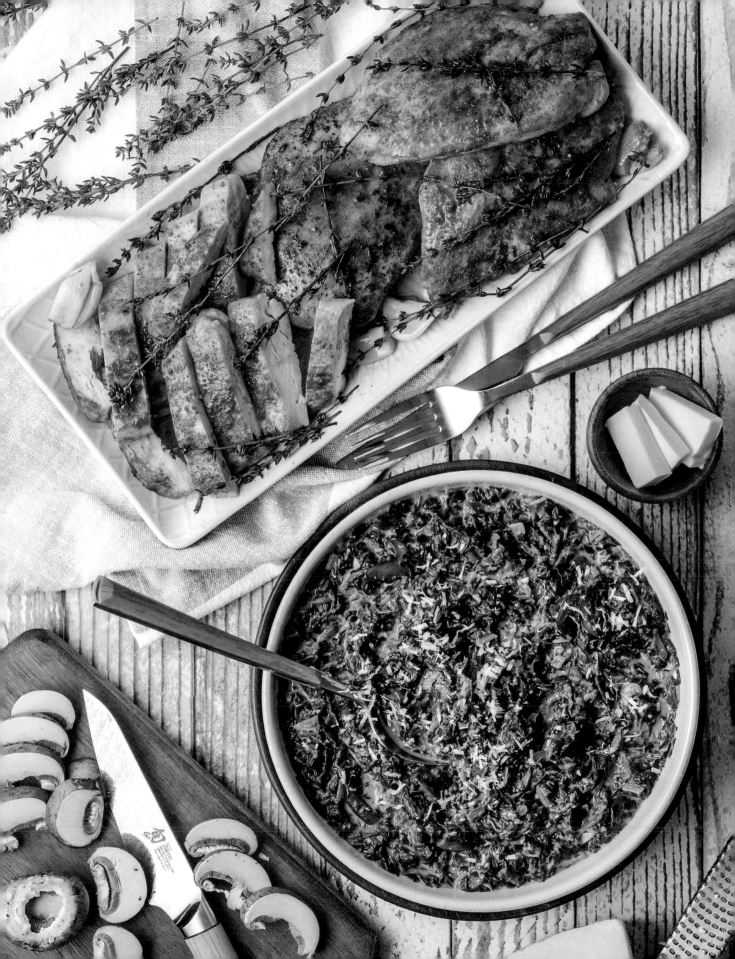

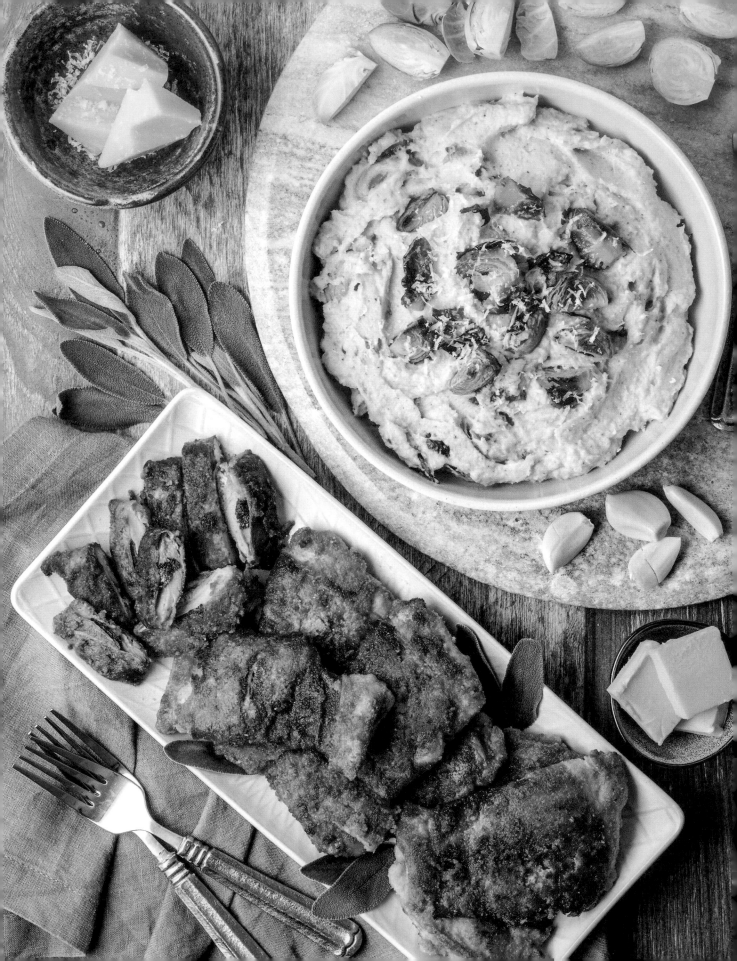

PREP TIME: **20 MINUTES** • COOKING TIME: **45 MINUTES** • MAKES: **5 MEALS**

CHICKEN SALTIMBOCCA
WITH GARLICKY ROASTED MASH

This recipe is all about taking your favorite comfort foods and making them keto. Almond flour–dusted chicken thighs wrapped in prosciutto and sage served with roasted cauliflower and brussels sprouts mash. Big time comfort, big time flavors.

 To watch the video tutorial for this recipe, search "FlavCity saltimbocca" on YouTube.

FOR THE MASH:
- 1 large head cauliflower
- ¾ pound brussels sprouts
- ½ teaspoon dried thyme
- ¼ cup heavy cream
- 1 tablespoon grass-fed unsalted butter
- ¼ cup grated Parmesan cheese
- 1 clove garlic
- Avocado oil
- Kosher salt and fresh pepper

FOR THE CHICKEN:
- 10 four-ounce chicken thighs, boneless and skinless
- 10 slices of prosciutto
- 10 sage leaves
- ½ cup almond flour
- Olive or avocado oil
- Kosher salt and fresh pepper

For the mash, preheat your oven to 425°F. Cut the cauliflower into large bite-size florets and place them on a sheet tray. Slice a small sliver from the root end of the brussels sprouts and then cut them in half lengthwise. Place the sprouts on the same sheet tray and season everything with 2 tablespoons of oil, dried thyme, 1 teaspoon of salt, and a few cracks of pepper. Give the pan a good shake and roast in the oven for 30–35 minutes until the veggies are charred in spots. Start to warm the cream over the lowest heat setting and add more than ¼ cup just in case you need it. Once veggies are ready, move on to the next step below using the blender. You want to do this while the veggies are hot.

While the veggies are roasting, **start on the chicken**. Season both sides of the thighs with a small amount of salt and pepper; the prosciutto is salty, so don't overdo it. Place a piece of prosciutto on a plastic cutting board, place the chicken thigh in the middle and then put one sage leaf in the center of the thigh. Wrap the prosciutto around the chicken tightly and repeat with remaining thighs.

Place the almond flour in a small baking dish or bowl and season with ¼ teaspoon of salt and a few cracks of pepper, mix well. Add the chicken to the almond flour, press down, flip, and repeat, making sure both sides are covered. Place chicken on a platter or on a wire rack set over a sheet tray. Repeat with remaining chicken. Preheat a large non-stick pan just above medium heat along with enough oil to coat the pan. Once the oil is hot, add half of the thighs to the pan. If the chicken does not sizzle right away, wait until it gets hotter. Cook chicken for 5 minutes, or until golden and crispy on the first side. Flip and repeat. The goal is to crisp the prosciutto while cooking the chicken all the way through, so adjust the heat if needed. Repeat with the second batch of chicken and set aside.

When the veggies come out of the oven, add only the cauliflower to the blender along with the warm cream, Parmesan, butter, and grate the clove of garlic using a microplane or fine grater. Blend on high speed until smooth—you may need to add more cream if the mixture is too thick. You can use a potato masher if you don't have a blender. Check for seasoning, you may need more salt or cheese. Transfer the puree to a clean bowl, roughly chop the roasted brussels sprouts, and then add to the puree and mix well.

Serve the chicken with the puree and enjoy!

STORAGE AND REHEATING: Everything will last in the fridge for five days or can be frozen for two to three months. The best way to reheat everything is in a 350°F oven for 8–10 minutes uncovered. If using a microwave, cover the container with a wet paper towel and make sure not to overheat or the food will dry out.

MACROS

per serving of chicken (2 thighs per serving):
413 calories
1 gram of net carbs
2 grams of total carbs
20.7 grams of fat
55.5 grams of protein
1.4 grams of fiber

MACROS

per serving of mash (makes 5):
208 calories
6.6 grams of net carbs
12.1 grams of total carbs
14.5 grams of fat
7 grams of protein
6.6 grams of fiber

★★★★★

"I made it and it was delicious! The chicken had amazing flavor and was super tasty even reheated days later. The cauliflower mash was perfect. I'll be making it again soon, thanks Bobby!" —**Maria C.**

"I made this, and it turned out amazing! It was so good that I'm going to make it again. Loved it that much! Thanks Bobby." —**Christine A.**

"Ok, seriously, I love your recipes. This one is the second one I made, and it totally makes me feel like I am eating a gourmet meal. I am learning so much from watching the videos that you have on YouTube. Even if I fail at the keto diet (not likely just saying), I will have learned to prepare food at a whole new level. THANK YOU!!!!!!! Keep them coming:)" —**Debra M.**

PREP TIME: **20 MINUTES** • COOKING TIME: **1 HOUR** • MAKES: **5 MEALS**

PALEO

MY BEST
CURRY CHICKEN SALAD

I noticed a long time ago that most people shake some curry powder in their mayo and call it a day. Sorry my friends—I may not be from Mumbai, but I do know that you need to bloom the essential oils in a hot pan with fat. This will intensify the flavor of your spices to the next level and give this curry mayo the proper flavor it deserves. Jai ho!

 Tip

Once the chicken comes out of the pan and has cooled, you will have a tasty dilemma. You can either devour that salty, crispy chicken *chicharrones* (skins) or chop it up and add it to the salad. Either way, don't you dare throw it out!

To watch the video tutorial for this recipe, search "FlavCity curry chicken salad" on YouTube.

FOR THE CURRY CHICKEN SALAD:

- 10 chicken thighs, bone-in and skin on
- Juice of ½ lemon
- ¼ cup green onions, sliced
- 2 tablespoons fresh Italian parsley, chopped
- ½ cup celery, sliced
- ¼ cup walnuts, chopped and roasted (optional)
- Kosher salt and fresh pepper

FOR THE CURRY MAYO:

- ¼ cup red onion, finely diced
- 1 teaspoon peeled ginger, freshly grated
- 2 cloves garlic, minced
- 2 teaspoons yellow curry powder
- 1 teaspoon ground turmeric
- ¼ cup chicken stock/broth
- 1 cup full-fat, sugar-free mayonnaise
- Zest and juice of ½ lime
- 2–3 drops of liquid stevia
- Kosher salt and fresh pepper
- Olive oil

For the chicken salad, preheat your oven to 400°F. Allow the chicken thighs to come to room temperature for 20 minutes and pat dry with a paper towel. Season both sides with a generous pinch of salt and a few cracks of pepper. Place the chicken skin side up on a sheet tray and cook in the oven for 55–60 minutes.

Make the curry mayo by preheating a medium-size, non-stick pan just over medium heat along with 2 teaspoons of olive oil. Add the chopped onions along with ¼ teaspoon of salt and a couple cracks of pepper, cook for 7 minutes, stirring often. Peel the skin off the fresh ginger using a spoon and then grate it on your microplane zester until you have 1 teaspoon. Add the ginger and garlic to the onions and cook for 2 minutes. Add the curry powder and turmeric along with 1 teaspoon of oil and stir well. Allow the curry and turmeric to cook for 1 minute; this way the essential oils can bloom and the flavor will release. Add the chicken stock and cook for 2–3 minutes or until the mixture has thickened up. Take off the heat and let cool down for 5–10 minutes.

Add the mayo to a food processor or blender along with lime zest and juice, stevia, ¼ teaspoon salt, and a couple cracks of pepper. Add the slightly cooled-down curry mixture to the mayo and blend on high until everything is well incorporated. Check for seasoning as you may need more stevia or lime juice.

When the chicken is ready, allow it to cool for 5–10 minutes and then remove the skin. Use two forks to shred the meat off the bones, and then chop everything into small pieces. Transfer the chicken to large bowl and season with ½ teaspoon of salt, few cracks of pepper, and the juice of half a lemon. Pour on enough curry mayo to thoroughly coat and mix well. Add more curry mayo if needed. Add the green onions, parsley, celery, walnuts, and mix well. Check for seasoning as you may need a little more lemon juice to make the flavors pop.

Serve the chicken salad with my soft and cheesy pita bread, see recipe on page 165.

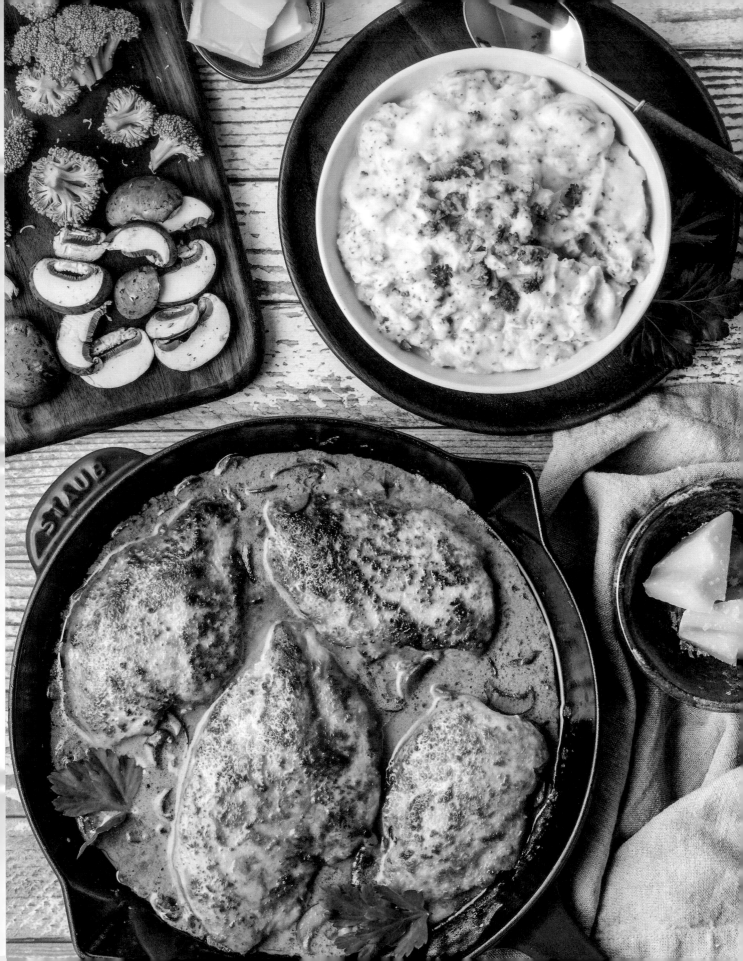

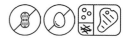

PREP TIME: **15 MINUTES** • COOKING TIME: **35 MINUTES** • MAKES: **5 MEALS**

CREAMY MUSHROOM CHICKEN
AND VEGGIE MASH

This is my keto take on comfort food. Nothing beats some creamy mushroom chicken with a big old scoop of mashed potatoes, but that's a no-no on the keto diet. Luckily, this whipped cauliflower mash is everything you want and more when trying to eat a low-carb diet.

 To watch the video tutorial for this recipe, search "FlavCity chicken and mushroom" on YouTube.

FOR THE CHICKEN:

- 1 teaspoon onion powder
- 1 teaspoon garlic powder
- 1 teaspoon fennel powder
- 5 boneless and skinless chicken breasts, pounded thin
- 10 ounces cremini mushrooms, sliced
- ½ cup chicken stock/broth
- ½ cup full-fat coconut milk
- Kosher salt and fresh pepper
- Olive or avocado oil

FOR THE MASH:

- 1 large head of cauliflower
- 4 cloves garlic, peeled
- 12 ounces broccoli florets
- 1 tablespoon unsalted grass-fed butter
- ¼ cup grated Parmesan or Pecorino Romano cheese
- Kosher salt and fresh pepper

Bring a medium-sized pot of water to a boil for the veggies.

Make the spice rub by combining the fennel, garlic, and onion powders in a small bowl, and mix well. Season both sides of the chicken with a generous pinch of the salt and spice rub. Let sit at room temperature for 20–30 minutes.

For the mash: Cut the cauliflower into large bite-size florets. Season the boiling water with 2 teaspoons of salt and boil the cauliflower florets along with the garlic for 7–9 minutes, or until you can mash the cauliflower with a fork. Make sure not to over-boil the cauliflower, as it will get too watery. Save the boiling water, strain the cauliflower and garlic, and place it in a blender. Add the broccoli florets to the boiling water, along with another pinch of salt and cook for 5–7 minutes, or until tender.

To finish the cauliflower mash, add the grated cheese, butter, ¼ teaspoon of salt, and a few cracks of pepper to the blender with the cauliflower. Blend until smooth and creamy and check for seasoning—you may need more salt.

Drain the broccoli and run under cold water for 30 seconds to stop the cooking process. Drain very well and then chop the broccoli. Add the chopped broccoli to the cauliflower mash and mix well. Check for seasoning and set aside.

For the chicken, preheat a large non-stick or cast-iron pan over medium-high heat for 2 minutes. Add 2 teaspoons of oil and wait 30 seconds to add the chicken to the pan. If your pan is not big enough, you will have to cook the chicken in two batches. Cook for 3–4 minutes or until the crust has a nice golden-brown color. Then flip and cook 2 minutes and remove from the pan. The chicken is still raw in the middle at this point. Add 1 teaspoon of oil to the pan along with the sliced mushrooms. Cook over medium heat for 10–12 minutes or until the mushrooms have wilted and have a nice golden color. Next, add ¼ teaspoon salt and a couple cracks of pepper. Add the coconut milk and chicken broth and stir well. Cook for 8–12 minutes or until the sauce has reduced by half. Check for seasoning, you will most likely need a pinch of salt and some pepper. Place the chicken back in the pan and cook for 5 minutes, or until the chicken is cooked through.

Serve the chicken with some mushroom sauce and veggie mash, enjoy!

While the chicken is cooking, **make the Alabama white BBQ sauce** by combining all the ingredients in a medium-sized bowl and whisking well. If the consistency is loose, add more mayo. Check for seasoning and adjust accordingly. The flavor should be tangy. Brush or spoon the white BBQ sauce all over the chicken, serve with the beans, and enjoy!

STORAGE AND REHEATING: Chicken should be stored in the fridge separately from the BBQ sauce, and both will keep for five days. You can freeze the chicken for two to three months, but not the sauce. The beans will keep for five days in the fridge or can be frozen for two to three months.

MACROS

per chicken thigh:
279 calories
0 carbs
17.5 grams of fat
28.3 grams of protein
0 fiber

MACROS

for all the BBQ sauce:
754 calories
0.89 grams of net carbs
1 gram of total carbs
83 grams of fat
1.2 grams of protein
0 fiber

MACROS

per serving of beans (makes 5):
190 calories
2.84 grams of net carbs
10.3 grams of total carbs
12.2 grams of fat
12.5 grams of protein
7.4 grams of fiber

★★★★★

"I made this tonight and it is AMAZING! Seriously delicious!! I foresee this being on repeat at my house. Thanks for a drool-worthy, healthy recipe." —**Britt D.**

"I made the chicken thighs last night and it was DELIIIISIOUS! The skin was super crispy and so flavorful. I gotta run and get some more smoked paprika too, cause I'm definitely going to repeat this recipe in the near future. Oh, and btw, my three-year-old licked his plate (never happens!). Thanks Bobby!" —**Yana**

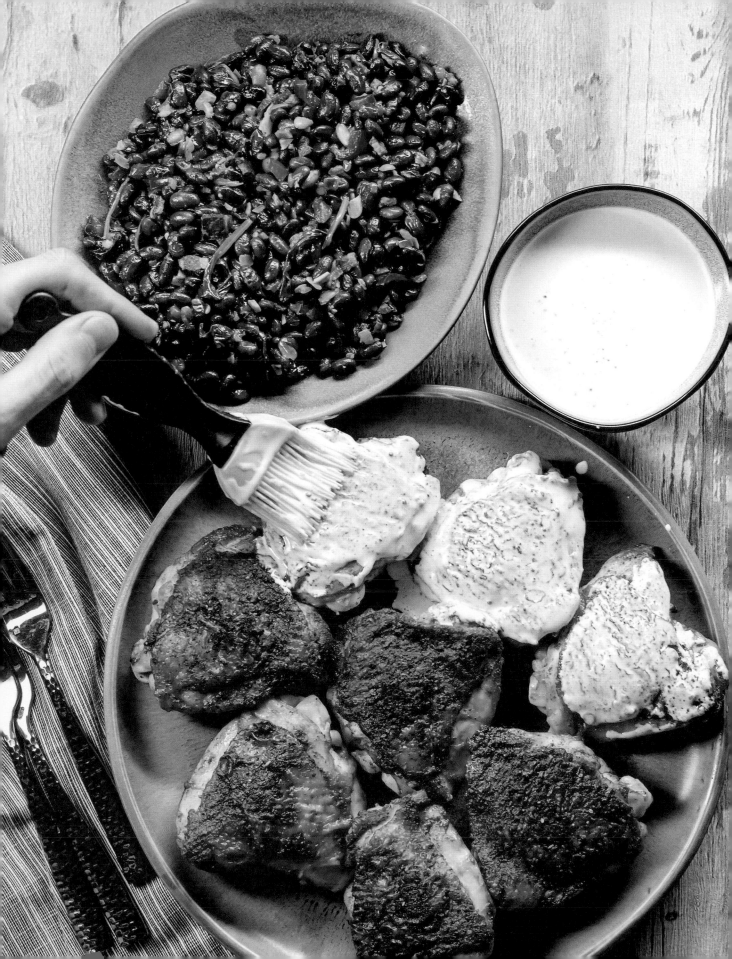

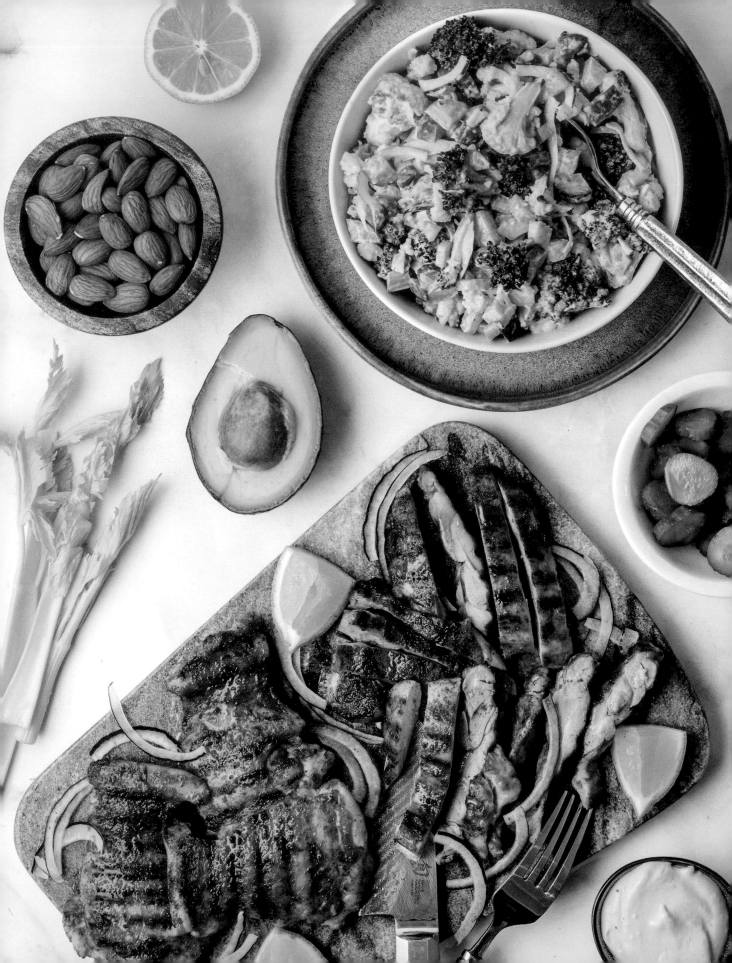

PREP TIME: **15 MINUTES** • COOK TIME: **40 MINUTES** • MAKES: **5 MEALS**

PALEO / WHOLE30

ROASTED VEGGIE SALAD
WITH FENNEL-SPICED CHICKEN THIGHS

One of the tops requests I get is for cold lunch recipes that you guys can take to work and school. This lunch recipe is so tasty, your coworkers will be seriously jealous and there is a good chance your lunch may go missing from the office fridge.

FOR THE CHICKEN:
- 1 heaping teaspoon ground coriander
- 1 heaping teaspoon fennel powder
- 1 heaping teaspoon sweet paprika
- 10 four-ounce chicken thighs, boneless and skinless
- Avocado oil
- Kosher salt and fresh pepper

FOR THE SALAD:
- 1 large head of cauliflower
- 12 ounces broccoli florets
- ¼ cup red onion, thinly sliced
- ½ cup pickles (no sugar added), chopped
- ½ cup celery, chopped
- ¼ cup almond, chopped
- 1–2 tablespoons fresh parsley, chopped
- Avocado oil
- Kosher salt and fresh pepper

FOR THE DRESSING:
- ¾ cup full-fat, sugar-free mayonnaise
- ½ a large avocado
- Juice of ½ lemon
- 1 clove of garlic, finely grated
- ½ teaspoon hot sauce, no sugar added
- ¼ teaspoon salt and fresh pepper

Make the spice rub for the chicken by combining the fennel, paprika, and coriander in a small bowl and mixing well. Season both sides of the chicken with a generous pinch of salt and the spice rub. Drizzle 1 tablespoon of oil over the chicken and allow to sit at room temperature for 20–30 minutes.

Start on the veggies by preheating the oven to 450°F. Cut the cauliflower into large bite-size florets. Place the florets on a sheet tray along with the broccoli florets and season with 1–2 tablespoons of oil, ¾ teaspoon salt, and a few cracks of pepper. Give the sheet pan a good shake and bake in the oven for 30–35 minutes, or until the veggies are well browned.

Make the dressing by combining everything in a blender or food processor, and blend to combine. You may need to add a splash of water if the dressing is too thick. Check for seasoning and adjust if necessary.

To finish the veggies, slice the red onions and place them in a small bowl of ice water for 5–30 minutes. This will remove the raw flavor. Once the cauliflower and broccoli are ready, add them to a large bowl along with the pickles, celery, almonds, parsley, and drained red onions. Add enough dressing to coat and mix well, adding more dressing if needed. Check for seasoning; you can add more dressing or lemon juice if needed.

To make the chicken, preheat a grill pan or cast-iron pan over medium-high heat for 2 minutes (non-stick pan will also work). Add 1 tablespoon of oil if using a flat-bottom pan and add half the chicken. Cook for 4–5 minutes, flip and repeat. If the chicken sticks to the grill pan, let it cook another minute or use a spatula to help flip. Repeat this step with the remaining chicken. Serve chicken with salad and enjoy!

STORAGE AND REHEATING: Everything will keep in the fridge for five days. You can freeze the chicken, but you can't freeze the veggie salad (will get watery and mushy). This meal prep is designed to be eaten cold.

MACROS

per serving of salad (makes 5):
125 calories
6.5 grams of net carbs
11.4 grams of total carbs
6.6 grams of fat
4.8 grams of protein
4.4 grams of fiber

MACROS

for all the dressing:
1361 calories
2.89 grams of net carbs
9.5 grams of total carbs
144 grams of fat
3.8 grams of protein
6.8 grams of fiber

MACROS

per serving of chicken (two thighs make one serving):
312 calories
0 carbs
13.6 grams of fat
48 grams of protein
0 fiber

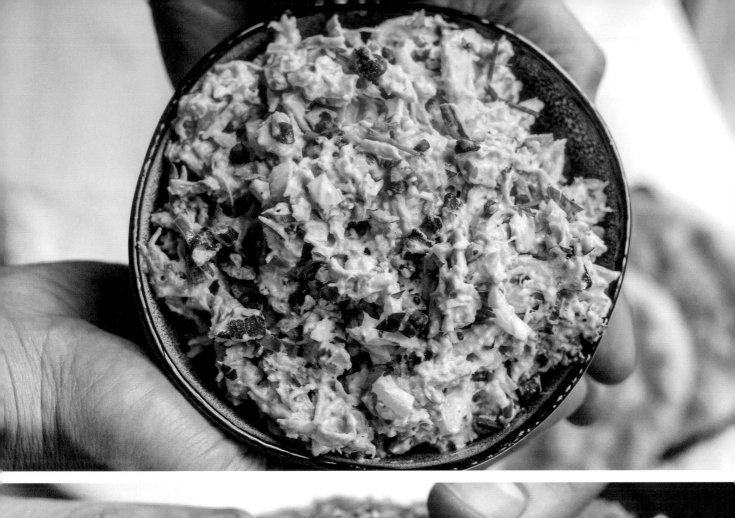
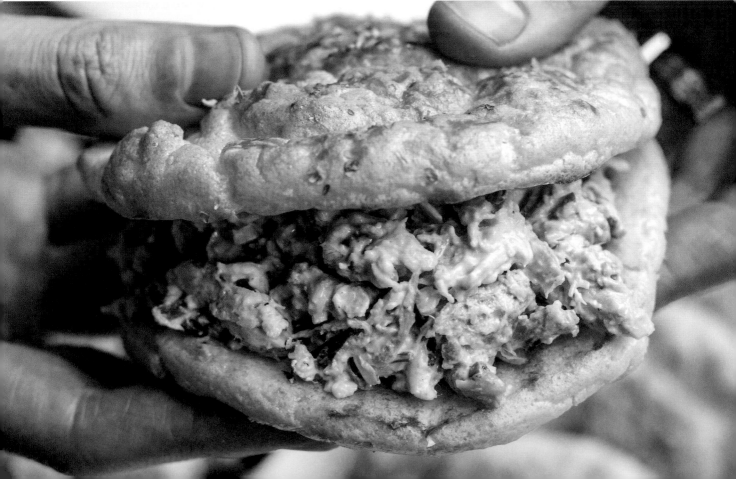

PREP TIME: **20 MINUTES** • COOKING TIME: **1½ HOURS** • MAKES: **5 MEALS**

ROASTED CHICKEN SALAD
WITH CLOUD BREAD

This meal prep recipe will make you eager for lunchtime at work or school. The chicken salad is juicy, crunchy, and loaded with flavor. The cloud bread is light and airy and makes the perfect sandwich for the salad.

Tip | For the cloud bread, you must beat the egg whites to stiff peaks and then gently fold in the egg and cream cheese mixture.

FOR THE CHICKEN SALAD:

- 10 chicken thighs, bone-in and skin on
- 4 slices sugar-free bacon, cooked and chopped
- Juice of ½ of lemon
- ¼ cup green onions
- 3 tablespoons fresh parsley, chopped
- ¼ cup chopped pecans, roasted if desired
- 1 cup celery, chopped
- Avocado or olive oil
- Kosher salt and fresh pepper

FOR THE DRESSING:

- 1 cup full-fat, sugar-free mayonnaise
- Juice of 1 lemon
- 1 teaspoon tamari soy sauce
- ½ teaspoon toasted sesame oil
- 1 teaspoon stone-ground or Dijon mustard
- 1 teaspoon hot sauce
- 1 teaspoon tahini
- ¼ teaspoon salt and a couple cracks of pepper

FOR THE CLOUD BREAD:

- See recipe on page 171

For the chicken, preheat oven to 400°F. Place the chicken thighs on a sheet tray and season with a drizzle of oil and a generous pinch of salt and a few cracks of pepper on both sides. Place the chicken skin side up and roast for 1 hour. You can also cook the bacon on a sheet tray for 15 minutes while the chicken roasts.

Make the dressing by combining everything in a medium-size bowl and whisking well. Check for seasoning: you want the flavor to be lemony and bold, so adjust if needed.

Once the chicken has cooled down for a few minutes, peel the skin off and use two forks to shred the meat off the bones. Then chop fine. Add the chicken to a large bowl and season it with ¼ teaspoon salt, a couple crack of pepper, and the juice of half a lemon. Mix well and then pour on all the dressing and mix very well. Add the green onions, parsley, pecans, celery, bacon, and mix very well. Check for seasoning you may need more lemon juice.

To make the cloud bread, see recipe on page 171.

Serve the chicken salad with the cloud bread and enjoy!

STORAGE AND REHEATING: The chicken salad will last in the fridge for five days but can't be frozen. The cloud bread should be cooled down and stored in a zip-top bag in the fridge for four or five days. It can also be frozen and reheated in a warm oven.

MACROS

per serving of chicken salad (makes 5):
702 calories
1.27 grams of net carbs
2.5 grams of total carbs
57.5 grams of fat
40 grams of protein
0.6 grams of fiber

MACROS

per cloud bread (makes 8):
93 calories
0.74 grams of net and total carbs
9.6 grams of fat
5.5 grams of protein
0.6 grams of fiber

★★★★★

"Oh em gee! I'm amazed with this recipe!! The cloud bread just melts and the chicken salad...yuuuuuuum!!! Loved the chicken "chicharrones"!! I totally can eat this for days! DELICIOUS!!" —**Julia**

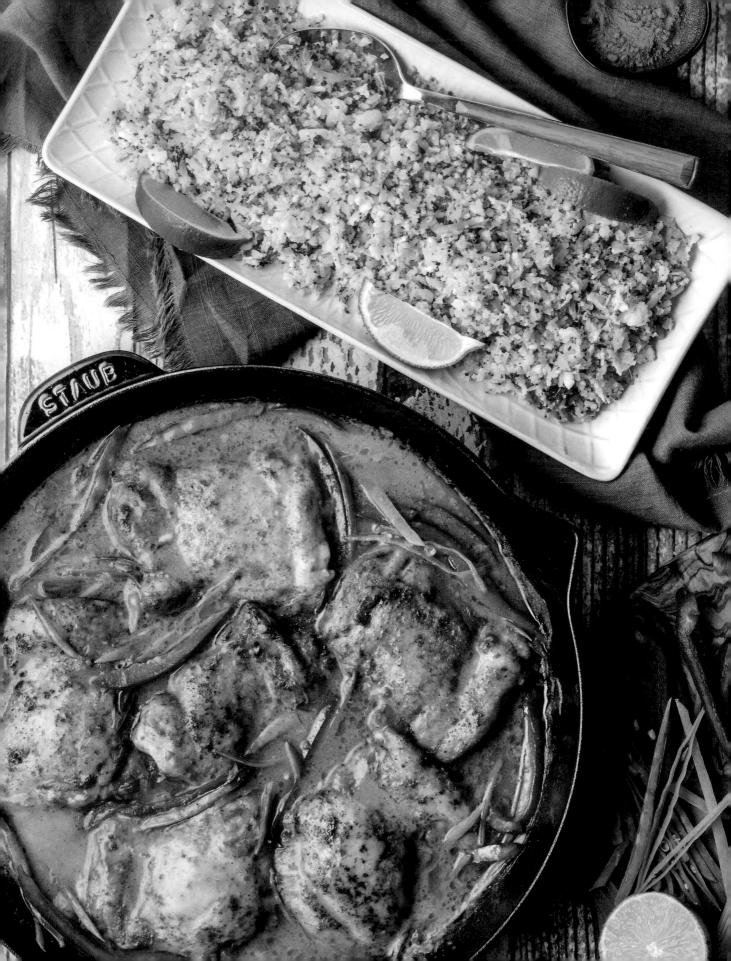

PREP TIME: **15 MINUTES** • COOKING TIME: **20 MINUTES** • MAKES: **5 MEALS**

PALEO / WHOLE30

ONE-PAN
COCONUT CURRY CHICKEN
WITH VEGGIE RICE

Only five fresh ingredients and two pans are needed for this recipe. Who said meal prepping had to be hard!? I love the flavor and creamy texture of this curry sauce. It's great for spooning over the veggie rice or going directly in your pie hole.

Tip
To make your life easier, you can buy cauliflower and broccoli rice from the store for this recipe. Buy the pre-grated one in the produce section instead of the frozen one, as the texture gets mushy when frozen.

You Tube
To watch the video tutorial for this recipe, search "FlavCity curry chicken" on YouTube.

INGREDIENTS:

- 10 four-ounce chicken thighs, boneless and skinless
- 2 teaspoons curry powder, like madras or moochi
- 1 teaspoon turmeric powder
- 1 13.5 oz can of full-fat coconut milk
- Juice of 1–2 limes
- 1 cup snow peas, thinly sliced at an angle
- 1 red bell pepper, sliced and halved
- 5 cups total of cauliflower and broccoli rice
- Avocado or coconut oil
- Kosher salt and fresh pepper

MACROS

per serving of chicken & rice
484 calories
6.1 grams of net carbs
9.1 grams of total carbs
27.1 grams of fat
47.9 grams of protein
3 grams of fiber

Make the chicken: Season both sides of the chicken with a generous pinch of curry powder and salt and let sit at room temperature for 20 minutes. Preheat a large cast-iron pan just below high heat with 2 teaspoons of oil for 2 minutes. Add half of the chicken to the pan and cook for 3 minutes or until the chicken is nicely browned; then flip and repeat. Remove the first batch of chicken from the pan and repeat the process with the second batch. Remove and set aside.

Turn off the heat for 2 minutes. Then add 1 teaspoon of oil to the pan along with the curry and turmeric powder and stir well, making sure the curry powder doesn't burn. Put the heat back on medium and cook for 1 minute to bloom the essential oils in the powder. Then immediately add the coconut milk and stir very well. Season the milk with the juice of half a lime, ¼ teaspoon of salt and a few cracks or pepper. Add the chicken back to the pan and bring to a simmer. Cook for 10 minutes with a lid or sheet pan covering the pan. Take the lid off, add the snow peas and peppers, and cook another 5 minutes or until the coconut milk has reduced by half. Check for seasoning as you may need more salt and/or lime juice. Take off the heat and set aside.

While the chicken is cooking, **make the veggie rice** by preheating a large non-stick pan over medium heat with 2 teaspoons of oil. Add the veggie rice and season ½ a teaspoon of salt and a few cracks of pepper. Mix well, place a lid on the pan, and cook for 5–7 minutes or until the veggies are tender and don't have a raw flavor. Add the juice of half a lime and check for seasoning. Remove from heat.

Serve the rice with chicken, veggies, and sauce and enjoy!

STORAGE AND REHEATING: Everything will keep in the fridge for five days, but only the chicken can be frozen for two to three months. Thaw and reheat in a 350°F oven for 7–10 minutes. If using the microwave, take lid off, cover with a wet paper towel, and reheat making sure not to heat too long or too hot or the chicken will dry out.

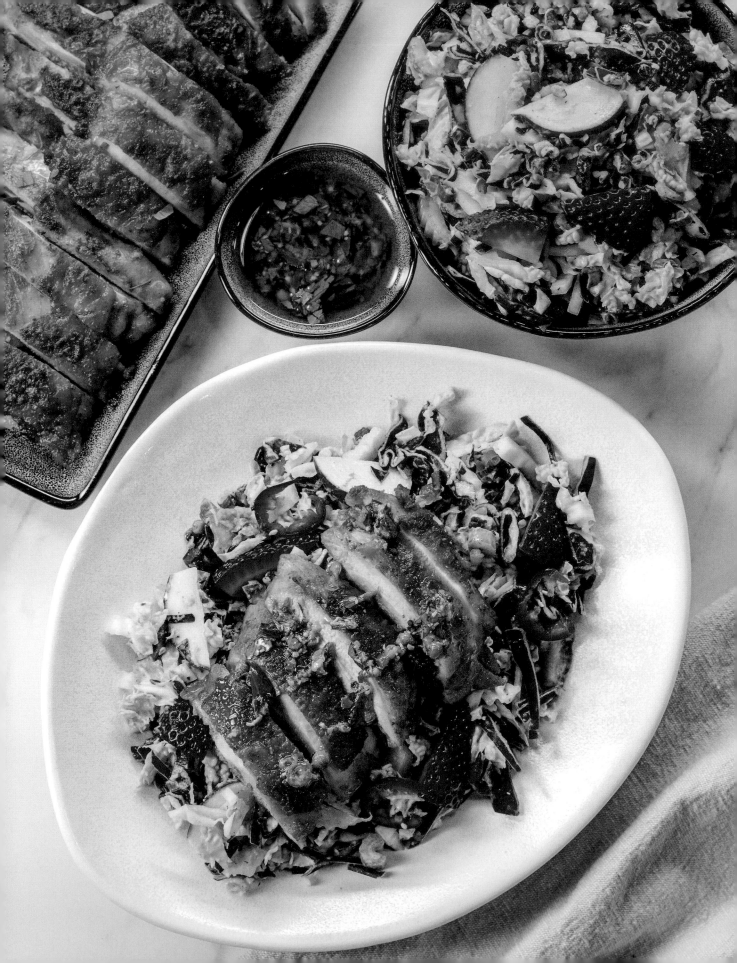

PREP TIME: **20 MINUTES** • COOK TIME: **35 MINUTES** • MAKES: **5 MEALS**

PALEO / WHOLE30

CRISPY CHICKEN THIGHS
WITH RED CABBAGE CRUNCH SLAW

The only thing better than juicy chicken meat is crispy skin. Luckily, this meal prep recipe has both, combined with a fresh and zippy salsa verde and a creamy cabbage slaw that will make it taste like summer all year round.

FOR THE CHICKEN:
- 1½ teaspoons smoked paprika
- 1½ teaspoons turmeric
- 10 chicken thighs, skin on and boneless
- Kosher salt
- Avocado oil

FOR THE SALSA VERDE:
- ¼ cup extra virgin olive oil
- 1 teaspoon fresh chopped parsley
- Zest and juice of ½ lemon
- 1 teaspoon capers, drained and minced
- 1 clove garlic, grated
- 1 teaspoon Dijon or stone-ground mustard
- ¼ teaspoon red pepper flakes or ½ a red chili, minced
- ⅛ teaspoon salt and one crack of black pepper

FOR THE COLESLAW:
- ½ head red cabbage
- ½ head Napa cabbage
- 1 cup celery, thinly sliced
- 4 radishes, thinly sliced
- ¼ cup chopped pecans, roasted if desired
- 3 tablespoons green onions, sliced
- ½ cup sliced strawberries
- ¼ cup tahini
- 2–3 tablespoons water
- Zest and juice of ½ lemon
- 1 clove garlic, grated
- ¼ teaspoon salt and a couple cracks of pepper

 Tip Ask the produce person to cut a head of cabbage in half for you; they will be happy to do it. If you want to be lazy, just buy a large bag of slaw mix. Trader Joe's has one called the crunch-a-ferious kale crunch salad, I love it! #TeamCrunch

 Tip Ask the butcher at the meat counter to take the bones out of the chicken thighs for you. Save those bones for soup and stock.

 To watch the video tutorial for this recipe, search "FlavCity keto chicken and slaw" on YouTube.

Make the spice rub for the chicken by combining the smoked paprika and turmeric in a small bowl and mix well. Season both sides of the chicken with a generous pinch of salt and the spice rub, along with a drizzle of oil. Rub the spices all around. Preheat two large pans (or use one, but you will have to cook in two batches) just below medium-high heat. Allow the pans to heat for two minutes (cast-iron is best, but non-stick will also work), and then add 1 tablespoon of oil and allow that to heat for 30 seconds before putting the chicken in skin side down. Allow to cook undisturbed for 5–6 minutes, or until the skin is well browned and crispy. Flip the chicken over, reduce heat to medium, and allow to cook another 3 minutes, or until the chicken is cooked through. (You may need to cut a piece in half to check.) Remove chicken, cover very loosely with foil, and set aside.

Make the salsa verde by combining all ingredients in a small bowl and mixing well. Check for seasoning; you want the flavor to be bright and lemony. Set aside.

Make the slaw by thinly slicing both half-heads of cabbage and adding them to a large bowl, along with the remaining ingredients up through the strawberries.

Make the dressing by adding the remaining ingredients to a small bowl along with enough water to make the consistency pourable. Check for seasoning; you may need more lemon juice. Wait until right before you are ready to serve to dress the slaw, and add ¼ teaspoon salt and a couple cracks of pepper. Mix well and, if you think it needs more dressing, make some more.

Serve the chicken with some salsa verde on top and a side of slaw, enjoy!

STORAGE AND REHEATING: Everything will keep in the fridge for five days, but you have to keep the dressing separate from the slaw and only dress it the morning of the day you want to enjoy it. You can freeze the chicken for two to three months but can't freeze the salsa verde or slaw.

MACROS

per piece of chicken (makes 10):
290 calories
0 grams of carbs
18.8 grams of fat
28.2 grams of protein
0 fiber

MACROS

for all the salsa verde:
501 calories
0.89 grams of net carbs
1 total grams of carbs
56 grams of fat
0 protein
0 fiber

MACROS

per serving of slaw (makes 5):
190 calories
7.03 grams of net carbs
12.02 grams of total carbs
14.27 grams of fat
5.9 grams of protein
5.1 grams of fiber

 ★★★★★

"Just made this meal for dinner and it's definitely a five-star meal from any restaurant made right in my kitchen. Thank you for the recipe!" —**Kristina**

"This was fantastic! My husband is on keto and I am mostly vegan (but I have salmon or shrimp here and there), so tonight I made this dish and substituted shrimp for myself! Everything turned out great. I am always nervous about making chicken or meat because I can't taste it, but my husband absolutely loved it! And that tahini dressing was soooo amazing! Thanks again for this amazingly easy yet flavorful recipe!" —**Nessa**

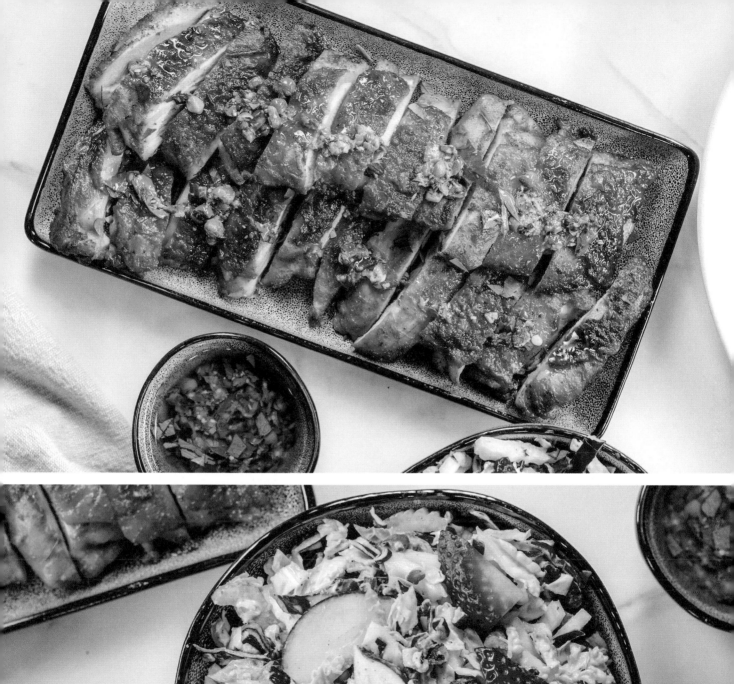
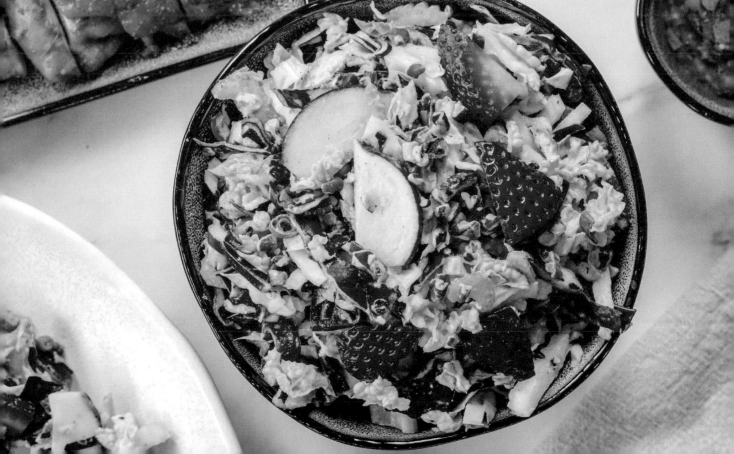

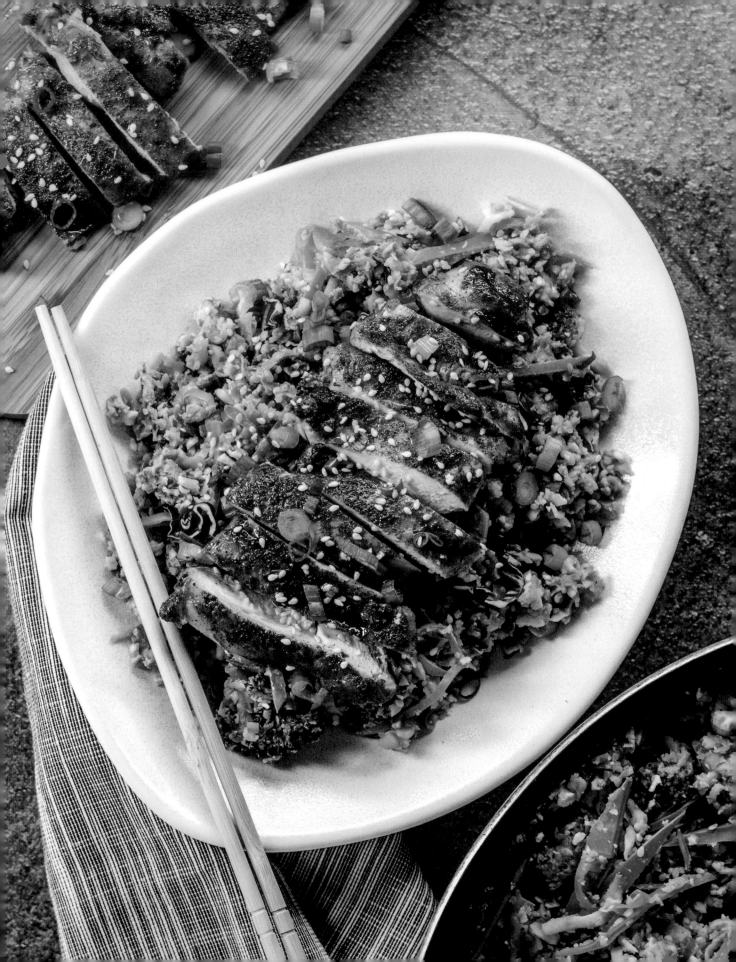

PREP TIME: **20 MINUTES** • COOKING TIME: **25 MINUTES** • MAKES: **5 MEALS**

CHICKEN FRIED CAULIFLOWER RICE

My favorite part of this cauliflower fried rice is the soft scrambled eggs running all throughout it. Paired with juicy, spice-crusted chicken thighs for the ultimate keto version of Asian takeout food.

Tip | Chinese five spice is like buying five spices for the price of one! It's great to keep in your pantry for a quick spice rub that will elevate chicken, steak, and pork.

You Tube | To watch the video tutorial for this recipe, search "FlavCity keto fried rice" on YouTube.

FOR THE CAULIFLOWER RICE:

- 5 cups of cauliflower rice, just about 1 large head
- ½ red onion, diced
- 2 cups of broccoli florets, cut in small bite-size pieces
- 1 cup snow peas, sliced thin on the diagonal
- ¾ cup red cabbage, shredded
- 3 cloves of garlic, minced
- 1 teaspoon fresh ginger, peeled and finely grated
- 3 eggs, beaten
- 1–2 tablespoons tamari soy sauce
- 1–2 teaspoons sambal oelek or sriracha
- 1 teaspoon toasted sesame oil
- ¼ cup green onions, finely sliced
- 1 teaspoon sesame seeds, toasted if desired
- Kosher salt
- Avocado oil

FOR THE CHICKEN:

- 10 boneless and skinless chicken thighs
- 1½ tablespoons Chinese five spice powder
- Kosher salt and fresh pepper
- Avocado oil

Season the chicken thighs with a generous pinch of salt and Chinese five spice on both sides along with 1 teaspoon of oil and rub the spices into the chicken. Allow to sit at room temperature for 20–30 minutes.

To make the cauliflower fried rice, use the large setting on a box grater to grate the cauliflower and set aside. Preheat a large, non-stick pan or wok over medium-high heat for 1 minute along with 1 tablespoon of oil. Add the onions, broccoli, ¼ teaspoon of salt, and a couple cracks of pepper. Cook for 5 minutes, stirring a few times. Add the snow peas, cabbage, garlic, ginger, and cook another 2–3 minutes, or until the broccoli has softened a bit. Whisk the eggs in a bowl, make a well in the middle of the pan with the veggies, and add the eggs. Mix the eggs until they look like a soft scramble and immediately add all the cauliflower rice and mix very well. Add the tamari, sambal or sriracha, toasted sesame oil, and mix well. Cook for 5 minutes, stirring very often. Check for seasoning—you may need more of the sauces. Turn the heat off the pan and add the green onions and sesame seeds, mix well, and transfer the cauliflower rice to a large bowl.

To cook the chicken, use the same pan and preheat it over medium-high heat for 2 minutes with 1 tablespoon of oil. Add half the chicken and cook for 4–5 minutes, flip and allow to cook another 3–4 minutes or until the chicken is cooked through. Once the chicken hits the pan, only flip it once—the goal is to create a beautiful crust and not disturb the chicken by moving it. Remove chicken from pan and cook the second batch. If you overcrowd the pan, the chicken won't sear and get a nice crust.

Serve the chicken with the cauliflower fried rice and enjoy!

STORAGE AND REHEATING: Everything will last in the fridge for five days. Only the chicken can be frozen for two to three months. To reheat, the preferred method is in a 350°F oven for 7–10 minutes. If using a microwave, cover the container with a wet paper towel and make sure not to overheat or the chicken will dry out.

MACROS

per serving of fried rice (makes 5):
146 calories
10.7 grams of net carbs
16.9 grams of total carbs
6.2 grams of fat
8.7 grams of protein
6.1 grams of fiber

MACROS

per chicken thigh (makes 10):
160 calories
0 carbs
8 grams of fat
24 grams of protein
0 fiber

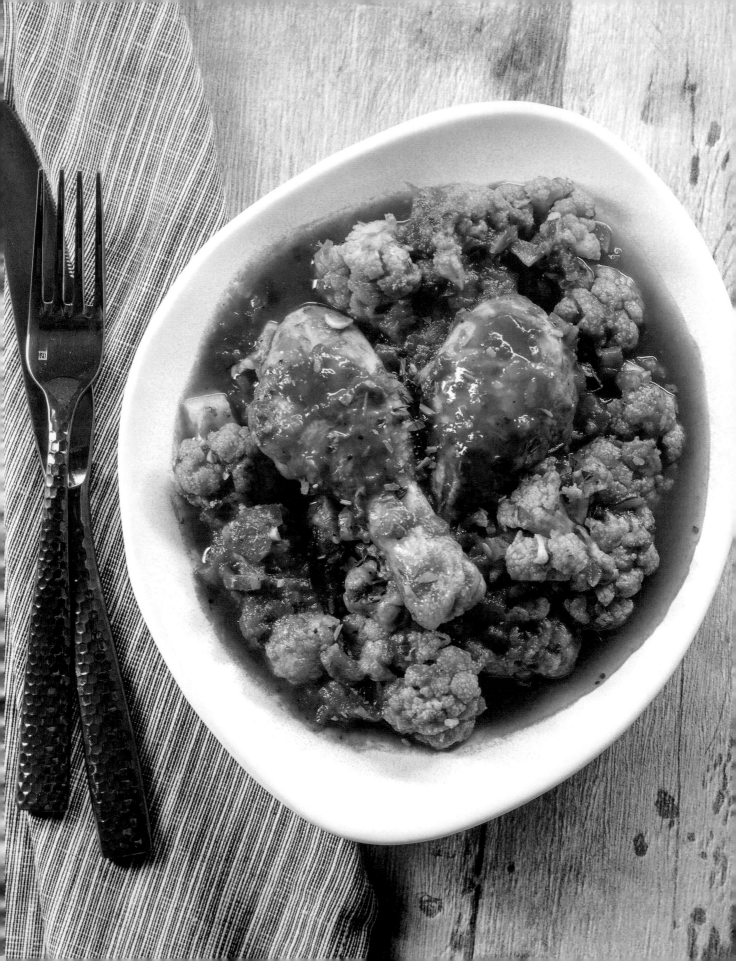

PREP TIME: **25 MINUTES** • COOKING TIME: **35 MINUTES** • MAKES: **5 MEALS**

PALEO

PRESSURE COOKER CHICKEN CACCIATORE
WITH CAULIFLOWER

This recipe is all about comfort food in a hurry. I was late to the electric pressure cooker party, but I now see what all the fuss is about. The chicken gets incredibly tender and falls off the bone in only 10 minutes of cooking time.

 Tip | You can make this recipe on the stovetop if you don't have an electric pressure cooker. Follow the same steps and gently simmer the chicken for 1–1½ hours with the lid on the pot. Remove chicken and cook the cauliflower florets until tender, about 10–15 minutes.

 Tip | Also, it's ok to cook with a bit of wine on keto, ¼ cup only has 1.5 total carbs.

 You Tube | To watch the video tutorial for this recipe, search "FlavCity chicken cacciatore" on YouTube.

INGREDIENTS:

- 10 chicken drumsticks
- ½ onion, chopped
- 2 stalks of celery, diced
- 1 medium zucchini, chopped
- ½ teaspoon dried oregano
- 3 cloves garlic, minced
- 2 tablespoons tomato paste
- ¼ cup white wine
- ¾ cup chicken stock/broth
- 1 fourteen-ounce can crushed tomatoes
- 1 bay leaf
- 1 head of cauliflower, cut into florets
- 1 tablespoon fresh Italian parsley, chopped
- Olive or avocado oil
- Kosher salt and fresh pepper

Preheat the electric pressure cooker to the highest sauté setting and season the chicken drumsticks with a generous pinch of salt and pepper on all side. Add 1 tablespoon of oil to the pot along with half of the chicken. There should be room for 5 drumsticks at one time. Sear for 3–4 minutes on both sides or until golden brown. Remove chicken from pot and sear the second batch.

Turn the heat down to the medium sauté setting and add another 2 teaspoons of oil to the pot along with the onions, celery, zucchini, oregano, ½ teaspoon salt, and a few cracks of pepper. Mix well and cook for 10 minutes. Add the garlic and cook for 2 minutes. Add the tomato paste and cook for one minute and then add the chicken back to the pot along with the wine, chicken broth, can of tomatoes, bay leaf, ½ teaspoon salt, and a few cracks of pepper. Mix well, place the lid on the electric pressure cooker, and set to pressure cook on high for 10 minutes.

After 10 minutes of cook time, let the electric pressure cooker sit for 10 minutes and then release the steam manually. Remove the chicken and add the cauliflower florets to the pot with the sauce and pressure cook on high for zero minutes. Release the steam and remove the cauliflower. Cooking the cauliflower any longer will make it mushy.

Serve the chicken cacciatore with the cauliflower, spoon some sauce over and garnish with parsley, and enjoy!

STORAGE AND REHEATING: Everything will keep in the fridge for five days or can be frozen for two to three months. Reheat in a 350°F oven for 7–10 minutes or cover the container with a wet paper towel and reheat in the microwave.

MACROS

per serving (makes 5):
433 calories
8.5 grams of net carbs
11.7 grams of total carbs
14.7 grams of fat
31 grams of protein
5.1 grams of net carbs

 ★★★★★

"That cacciatore was a hit...I had to make two pots, one keto friendly and the other I put potatoes in. Thanks again!!!!!" —**Gene N.**

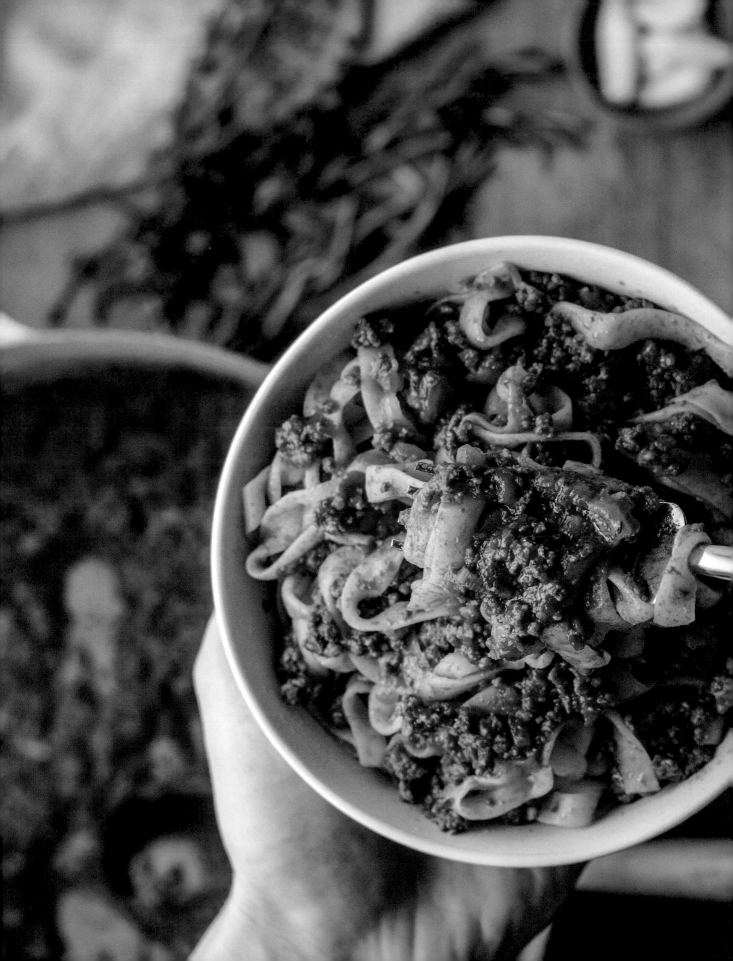

PASTA LA VISTA, BABY!

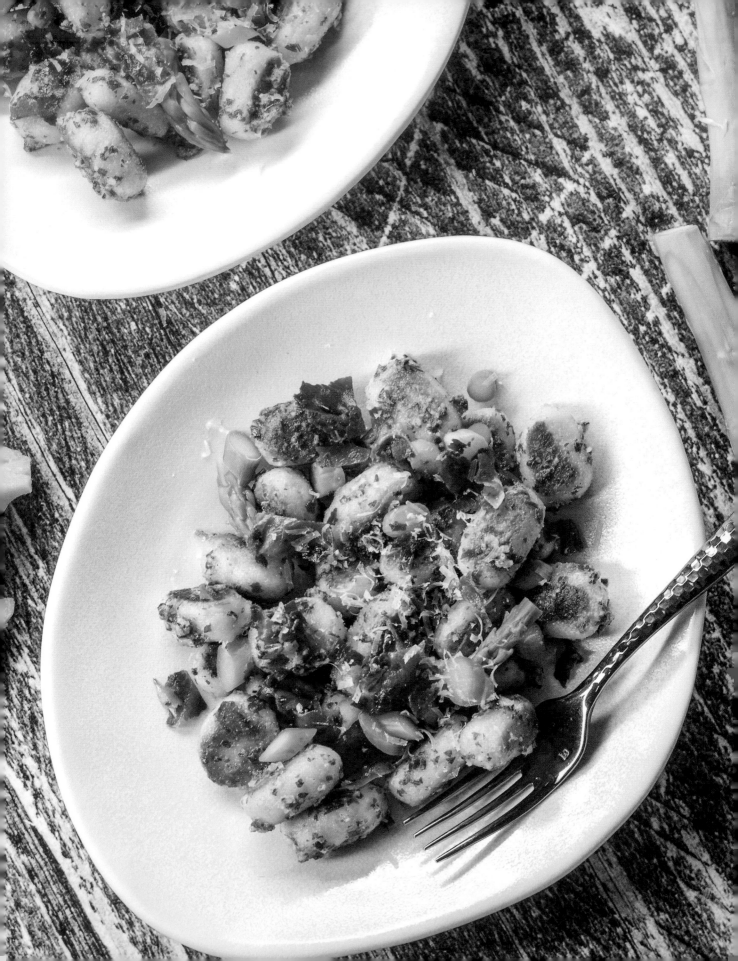

PREP TIME: **25 MINUTES** • COOKING TIME: **10 MINUTES** • MAKES: **4 SERVINGS**

GNOCCHI WITH PESTO SAUCE
AND CRISPY PROSCIUTTO

I asked Dessi to come up with a keto gnocchi recipe, and she totally blew my mind! These almond flour gnocchi taste just like the real thing, and, when tossed in pesto sauce and topped with crispy prosciutto, you won't even miss all those carbs.

 Tip | Follow the gnocchi instructions exactly as they are. These gnocchi are a bit fickle to make but totally worth the effort.

 | To watch the video tutorial for this recipe, search "FlavCity keto gnocchi" on YouTube.

FOR THE GNOCCHI:
- 4 eggs
- 4 teaspoons baking powder
- ¾ teaspoon kosher salt
- 4 cups (12 oz) of finely shredded, low-moisture mozzarella cheese
- 3 cups blanched almond flour

FOR THE PESTO:
- 1 cup fresh basil
- 1 cup Italian flat leaf parsley
- 2 cloves of garlic
- Zest of ½ lemon and 1 tablespoon of lemon juice
- ⅓ cup pecans, roasted if desired
- ¼ cup extra virgin olive oil
- ¼ cup fresh grated Parmesan or Pecorino Romano cheese
- ¼ teaspoon kosher salt
- Couple cracks fresh pepper

FOR THE FINAL TOUCHES:
- 12 ounces asparagus
- 4 slices of prosciutto

For the gnocchi, beat the eggs in a large bowl, add the salt and baking powder, and mix well. Add the finely grated cheese and mix well with a spatula. Add the almond flour and mix well. Continue to mix the dough for 1–2 minutes using your hands or a pastry cutter. It's important to mix well so the cheese and almond flour get fully incorporated. Let the dough rest for 20 minutes at room temperature in a bowl. Cut the dough into 4 pieces, add a little almond flour to a plastic cutting board or on your countertop, and roll each piece of dough into a long sausage shape—you can cut the dough into two pieces if that makes it easier. Watch the video on YouTube to see how we do it. You want the dough to be about ¾ inch thick. Use a knife to cut the dough into roughly half-inch gnocchi pieces and then roll each one tightly and form into a gnocchi (football) shape. Repeat with remaining dough and place formed gnocchi on a platter and in the freezer for 15–20 minutes. After that, you can place them in a freezer bag and freeze for two months. Gnocchi must be frozen when cooked in boiling water.

Make the pesto by adding the basil, parsley, garlic, lemon zest and juice, pecans, salt, and pepper to a food processor and blend until everything is well combined—about 10–15 seconds. With the machine running, slowly add the olive oil and process until combined and very smooth. Add the cheese and process another 10 seconds. Turn the machine off and taste the pesto—it might need more cheese or lemon juice. If the consistency is a little dry, add 2–4 tablespoons more oil while the machine is running.

Make the crispy prosciutto by preheating a large non-stick pan (will use that pan for gnocchi later) just above medium heat. Add the sliced prosciutto and cook until crispy on both sides—about 5–6 minutes total. Remove and set aside.

Bring a large pot of water to boil for the gnocchi and asparagus. Cut the bottom end of the asparagus off, season the boiling water with 2 teaspoons of salt, and cook the asparagus for exactly one minute. Remove the asparagus (but **save** the boiling water) and run under ice cold water for 30 seconds. Set aside.

FOLLOW THESE INSTRUCTIONS EXACTLY FOR COOKING THE GNOCCHI.
Don't boil all the gnocchi at once. You need to work in four batches to

make sure they cook evenly and don't get smashed. Make sure the water is **not boiling**. It should be at a bare simmer. Otherwise, the gnocchi could fall apart.

Preheat the same pan used to cook the prosciutto over medium-high heat with 2 teaspoons of oil. Place a strainer in the water if you have it and add ¼ of the gnocchi. Cook for exactly 30 seconds, drain, and place in the hot pan and carefully cook for 1–2 minutes until nicely golden on both sides. Transfer gnocchi to a plate and repeat that process with the remaining gnocchi. I know it's a pain, but these gnocchi are very fragile. Once all the gnocchi are cooked, I find it best to return them to the pan over low heat and add as much of the pesto as desired and toss to coat for 30 seconds or until warmed through and coated nicely.

Toss gnocchi with sliced asparagus and crumble crispy prosciutto on top. Enjoy!

STORAGE AND REHEATING: The gnocchi will keep in the fridge for three days or can be frozen for two months. The best way to reheat is in a hot pan with more pesto. If using a microwave, cover the container with a wet paper towel and make sure not to overheat.

MACROS

per serving of gnocchi without pesto sauce (makes 4):
479 calories
9.3 grams of net carbs
17.2 grams of total carbs
55 grams of fat
36 grams of protein
7.9 grams of fiber

MACROS

for all the pesto sauce:
861 calories
4.4 grams of net carbs
10.7 grams of total carbs
89.1 grams of fat
13.1 grams of protein
5.8 grams of fiber

★★★★★

"This is the first recipe I've made twice on here. I also used the gnocchi 'dough' recipe to make a fairly decent keto-friendly pizza." —**Max**

"I am an old woman, and this is one of the best dishes I have ever made. Well worth the effort!! Followed directions and perfect the first time." —**Lisa**

PREP TIME: **15 MINUTES** • COOKING TIME: **60 MINUTES** • MAKES: **5 MEALS**

PALEO / WHOLE30

GREEK CHICKEN
WITH SPAGHETTI SQUASH PRIMAVERA

If you are going to eat a chicken breast, this is how you do it. Bone-in, skin on, and drenched in a lemony olive oil marinade that renders the chicken moist and tender. This will make you forget the days of dry, overcooked chicken breast! Oh, and the spaghetti squash is pretty gangster too.

 Tip | **First, roast the squash and then cook the chicken. I know it takes some time, but you don't want to cook both together in the oven because the moisture from the squash will affect the color of the chicken.**

FOR THE SPAGHETTI SQUASH:

- 7½ cups of cooked spaghetti squash, about 5½ pound raw squash
- ½ red onion, chopped
- 1 green bell pepper, thinly sliced
- 1 bulb of fennel, chopped
- 1 cup cherry tomatoes, halved
- 2 cloves of garlic, minced
- ½ red finger pepper, finely sliced or ½ teaspoon red pepper flakes
- Zest of 1 lemon
- Juice of ½ lemon
- 3 tablespoons freshly chopped Italian flat leaf parsley
- 3 tablespoons of chopped and toasted pecans
- Olive oil
- Kosher salt and fresh pepper

FOR THE CHICKEN:

- 5 bone-in chicken breasts
- 6 cloves of garlic, finely grated or chopped
- ½ teaspoon dried oregano
- ½ teaspoon thyme
- Zest of 2 lemons
- Juice of 2 lemons
- ¼ cup olive oil
- Kosher salt and fresh pepper

For the squash, preheat the oven to 400°F. Carefully cut the squash in half from top to bottom and scoop out the seeds. Place squash cut side up on a tin foil–lined sheet tray. Roast in the oven for 65–75 minutes. Don't add salt at this step because that will pull excess water to the surface and make the squash watery. You will know the squash is ready when a knife pierces deep into the flesh with ease; if it still feels hard, roast for another 15 minutes. Now would be a good time to start marinating the chicken below.

While the squash is roasting, preheat a large non-stick pan over medium heat with 1½ tablespoons of olive oil. Add the chopped onions, bell peppers, and fennel, along with ½ teaspoon of salt and a couple cracks of pepper. Cook for 10 minutes, stirring occasionally. Add the tomatoes, garlic, sliced chilies, and cook for another 4 minutes or until all the veggies have softened. Check for seasoning, you may need a small pinch of salt. Turn off the heat and set aside.

Once the squash has cooled down, use a large fork and rake the squash from top to bottom and add to a large bowl, along with the lemon zest, lemon juice, pecans, parsley, and ½ teaspoon of salt. Mix well, add the cook veggies and toss together. Check for seasoning and adjust if necessary.

Make the marinade for the chicken by combining the garlic, oregano, thyme, lemon zest and juice, and olive oil in a bowl. Whisk well to combine. Place the chicken breasts on a tin foil–lined sheet tray and pour on the marinade. Mix well to coat the chicken. Allow the chicken to sit at room temperature, skin side down, in the marinade for 20–30 minutes before baking in a 400°F oven. Season both sides with a generous pinch of salt and pepper, and cook skin side up for 45 minutes in the oven, or until the internal temperature reaches 155°F. Remove from oven and allow to rest 10 minutes before eating. Serve chicken with spaghetti squash and enjoy!

STORAGE AND REHEATING: Everything will last in the fridge for five days. The chicken can be frozen for two to three months, but the squash will get mushy if frozen. Reheat the squash and thawed chicken in a 350°F oven for 7–10 minutes. Make sure to drizzle a shot of olive oil over the chicken for added moisture while reheating. If using the microwave, make sure not to overheat or the chicken will dry out.

MACROS

per chicken breast:
308 calories
2 grams of net and total carbs
19 grams of fat
30 grams of protein
0 fiber

MACROS

per serving of squash (makes 5):
193 calories
15.8 grams of net carbs
21.2 grams of total carbs
12 grams of fat
3.1 grams of protein
5.9 grams of fiber

★★★★★

"Just got done making this meal for the week and I've got to say, it was great! I just found your YouTube channel last week. I've watched a couple of episodes and was very impressed with not only how healthy the meals were but how appetizing they looked. I've been cooking for the week for a while now to save money and eat healthier, so I'm looking forward to seeing more of your recipes. Thanks a lot, and keep them coming!" **—Augustus A.**

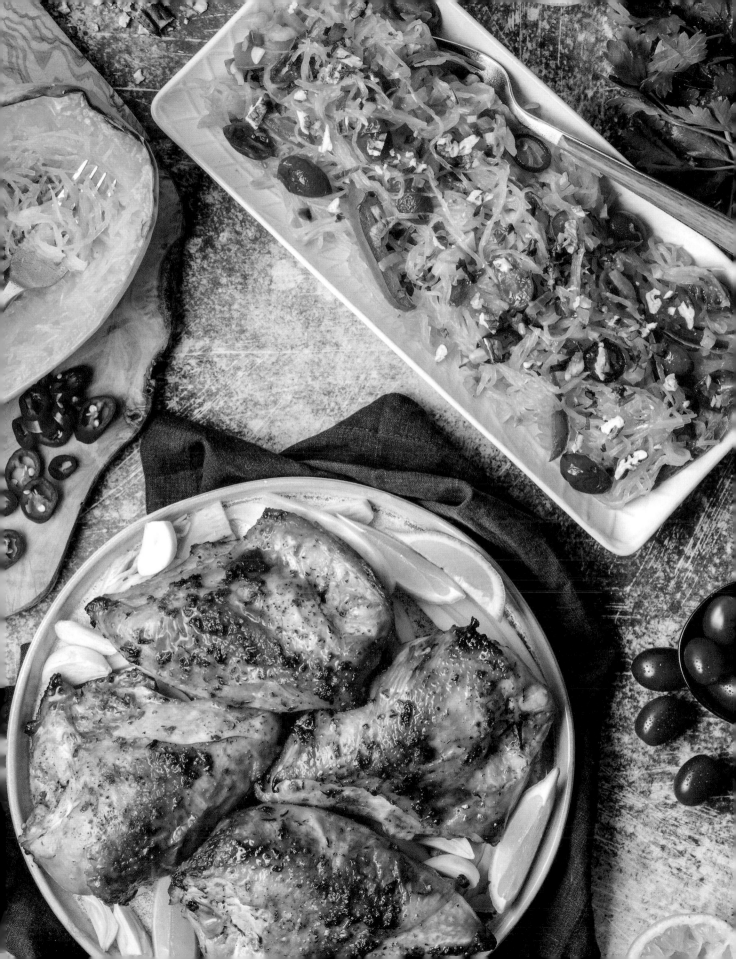

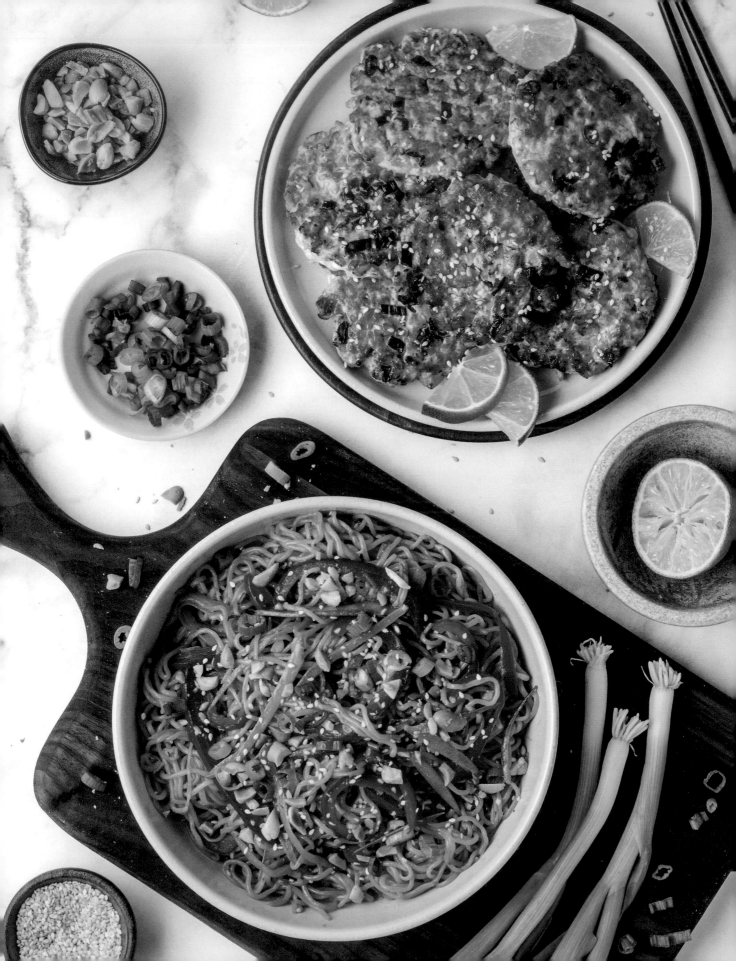

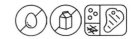

PREP TIME: **20 MINUTES** • COOKING TIME: **30 MINUTES** • MAKES: **5 MEALS**

ASIAN SALMON CAKES
AND NOODLE STIR-FRY

No need to break out your food processor for these salmon cakes. Just channel your inner iron chef and chop away. The stir-fry is a great way to get your noodle fix on the keto diet.

Tip | When buying salmon, ask the fishmonger to remove the skin for you, they will be more than happy to do it.

To watch the video tutorial for this recipe, search "FlavCity salmon stir fry" on YouTube.

FOR THE SALMON:
- 2 pounds of Atlantic salmon, skin removed
- 3 cloves garlic, finely grated
- 1½ teaspoons finely grated ginger
- 3 tablespoons green onions, sliced
- 1 teaspoon sesame seeds, toasted if desired
- Kosher salt and fresh pepper
- Avocado oil

FOR THE STIR-FRY:
- 2 pounds of shirataki noodles (pasta zero by Nasoya)
- 1 red bell pepper, sliced
- 1 cup snow peas, sliced on the angle
- 1–2 teaspoons sambal oelek or sriracha
- 2–3 tablespoons tamari soy sauce or coconut aminos
- 1 teaspoon toasted sesame oil
- Juice of ½ lime
- ¼ cup green onions, sliced
- 2 tablespoons unsalted peanuts, chopped
- Avocado oil

To prep the salmon cakes, use a plastic cutting board and cut the salmon into large cubes and then chop until the texture is fine. Transfer the salmon to a large bowl and add the grated garlic and ginger, green onions, 1 teaspoon salt, and a few cracks of pepper. Use your hands to thoroughly combine the mixture and then place in the fridge for at least 15 minutes so the mixture can chill.

Drain the noodles from their water and add them to a large non-stick pan set over medium-high heat. Cook for about 8–10 minutes or until most of the moisture is gone and the bottom of the pan looks white and cakey, stirring often. Spill the noodles on a cutting board and slice them a few times so they are not tangled together, then move noodles to a bowl. Preheat the same pan over medium-high heat with 2 teaspoons of oil for 1 minute. Add the red peppers and sliced snow peas and cook for 5 minutes, stirring often. Add the noodles back to the pan along with the sambal, tamari, sesame oil, the juice of half a lime and stir well. Cook for 1 minute and then check for seasoning. You will likely need more of the sauces, so adjust according to your taste. Cook for 2 more minutes, stirring often and turn off the heat. Add the green onions and peanuts and stir to combine. Remove noodles and set aside.

Cook the salmon cakes. Using the same pan, preheat over medium-high heat with ½ teaspoon oil for 2 minutes. Grab the salmon mixture from the fridge and use your hands to form large golf ball–size shapes. Place in the pan and use your hand to carefully pat the ball down into a patty. Place a total of 5 patties in the pan and use a fish spatula to press down and make the patties a little flatter. Cook for 4 minutes or until the first side is golden brown and flip and cook another 2–3 minutes. Remove from pan and repeat with the remaining salmon mixture.

Serve the fish cakes with some noodles and garnish with sesame seeds, and enjoy!

STORAGE AND REHEATING: The noodles will keep in the fridge for five days but can't be frozen. The salmon will keep in the fridge for three days or can be frozen for two months. Thaw and reheat salmon and noodles in a 350°F oven for 7–10 minutes. If using a microwave, cover the container with a wet paper towel and make sure not to overheat or the salmon will dry out.

MACROS

per salmon cake (makes 10):
135 calories
1.3 grams of net carbs
2 grams of total carbs
6.36 grams of fat
18 grams of protein
0 fiber

MACROS

per serving of stir-fry (makes 5):
75.2 calories
4 grams of net carbs
8.4 grams of total carbs
3.7 grams of fat
3.4 grams of protein
4.2 grams of fiber

★★★★★

"This is, hands down, the BEST keto meal I have had since starting almost one year ago. I have had quite a few fails with the shirataki noodles before, but now I doubt I'll ever make them any other way! The amazing flavor profile had every happy cylinder in my brain firing from the first bite. This recipe is bookmarked and definitely going into my regular meal rotation. Awesome job and keep up the fabulous work!!!" —**Cherissa W.**

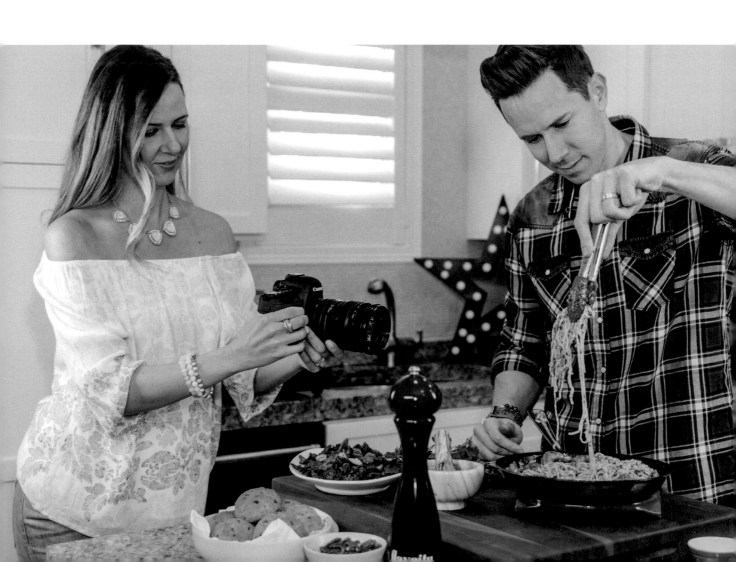

PREP TIME: **15 MINUTES** • COOKING TIME: **40 MINUTES** • MAKES: **5 MEALS**

RAMEN NOODLE SOUP
WITH PORK AND MUSHROOM WRAPS

There are a few epic ramen shops in Chicago, but we had to stop going because the MSG has a brutal effect on our bodies and the noodles are carb heavy. So, I came up with this quick and easy ramen recipe featuring my favorite shirataki noodles and paired it with lettuce wraps filled with juicy and fatty ground pork and mushrooms. Arigato gozaimashita!

 To watch the video tutorial for this recipe, search "FlavCity ramen" on YouTube.

FOR THE RAMEN:

- 4 ounces shitake mushrooms, sliced
- ½ cup chopped red onions
- 3 cloves garlic, minced
- 1 teaspoon freshly grated ginger
- 4 tablespoons miso paste
- 2 quarts beef stock/broth
- 1 teaspoon toasted sesame oil
- 2 tablespoons tamari soy sauce
- 1 teaspoon sambal oelek chili paste or sriracha
- 1 pound shirataki noodles (pasta zero by Nasoya)
- 1 soft-boiled egg, herbs, and chilies for garnish
- Kosher salt
- Avocado oil

FOR THE WRAPS:

- 10 ounces cremini or baby bella mushrooms
- ½ onion, chopped
- 1½ pounds ground pork
- 3 cloves garlic, minced
- 1 teaspoon fresh ginger, finely grated
- 2 teaspoons of sambal oelek chili paste or sriracha
- 3 tablespoons tamari soy sauce
- 1 teaspoon toasted sesame oil
- Lime juice
- 2 tablespoons unsalted and roasted peanuts, chopped
- 2 tablespoons green onions, finely sliced
- 2 heads of butter lettuce or romaine lettuce
- Avocado oil
- Kosher salt

For the ramen, cut the stems off the mushrooms and finely slice the top part. Preheat a soup pot over medium heat along with 1 tablespoon of oil. Add the mushrooms and onions, and cook for 10 minutes. Add the grated ginger and garlic, and cook 3 minutes. Add the miso paste, mix well, and cook for 1 minutes then add the beef broth. Raise the heat to high and add the sesame oil, tamari soy sauce, and chili sauce. Once the soup is boiling, reduce to a simmer and allow to cook for 20 minutes. Check for seasoning after 10 minutes; you may need more tamari or chili sambal, so adjust according to your preference. Drain and rinse the shirataki noodles and add them to the soup. Simmer another 5 minutes then turn the heat off. To make a ramen egg, bring a pot of water to a boil and cook the egg for 8 minutes, then immediately move to a bowl of ice water to stop the cooking process. Peel the egg and set aside.

For the lettuce wraps, remove them stems from the mushrooms and chop the mushroom caps into small pieces. Preheat a large pan just above medium heat for 2 minutes along with 1 tablespoon of oil. Add the onions and mushrooms and cook for 8–10 minutes. Raise the heat to medium-high and add the pork and use a wooden spoon or spatula to break the pork into small pieces. Cook for 3 minutes then add the garlic, ginger, and ¼ teaspoon of salt. Continue cooking a few more minutes until most of the pink color is gone from the pork and lower the heat to low. Add the sambal, tamari, sesame oil, a little squeeze of lime juice, and mix well. Turn the heat off the pan once the pork is cooked through and check for seasoning. You will most likely need more tamari or chili paste. Add the peanuts and green onions, then mix well and set aside.

To assemble the lettuce wraps, fill individual cups of lettuce with the pork mixture and garnish with more peanuts and green onions. To serve the ramen, fill a bowl and top with sliced chilies, green onions, a boiled egg cut in half, or any toppings you want. Enjoy!

STORAGE AND REHEATING: The lettuce wrap mixture and soup will last in the fridge for five days or can be frozen for two to three months. Reheat the soup on the stovetop and the pork mixture in a hot pan. If using the microwave for the pork mixture, cover the container with a wet paper towel and make sure not to overheat or the pork will get dry.

MACROS

per serving of ramen (makes 5):
88 calories
6.5 grams of net carbs
9.5 grams of total carbs
4 grams of fat
5.5 grams of protein
3.1 grams of fiber

MACROS

per serving of wraps (makes 5):
436 calories
4.1 grams of net carbs
5.3 grams of total carbs
34.3 grams of fat
26.6 grams of protein
1.2 grams of fiber

★★★★★

"Made this for dinner this evening. Easy to prepare and really tasty. Thank you for yet another great recipe, Bobby." —**Stephanie C.**

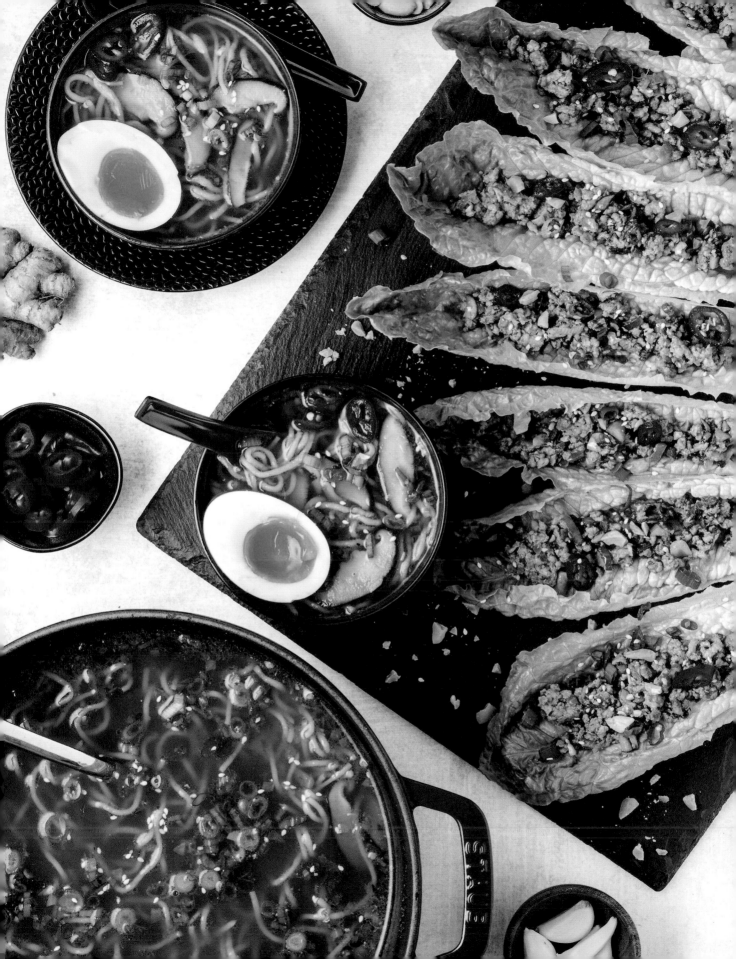

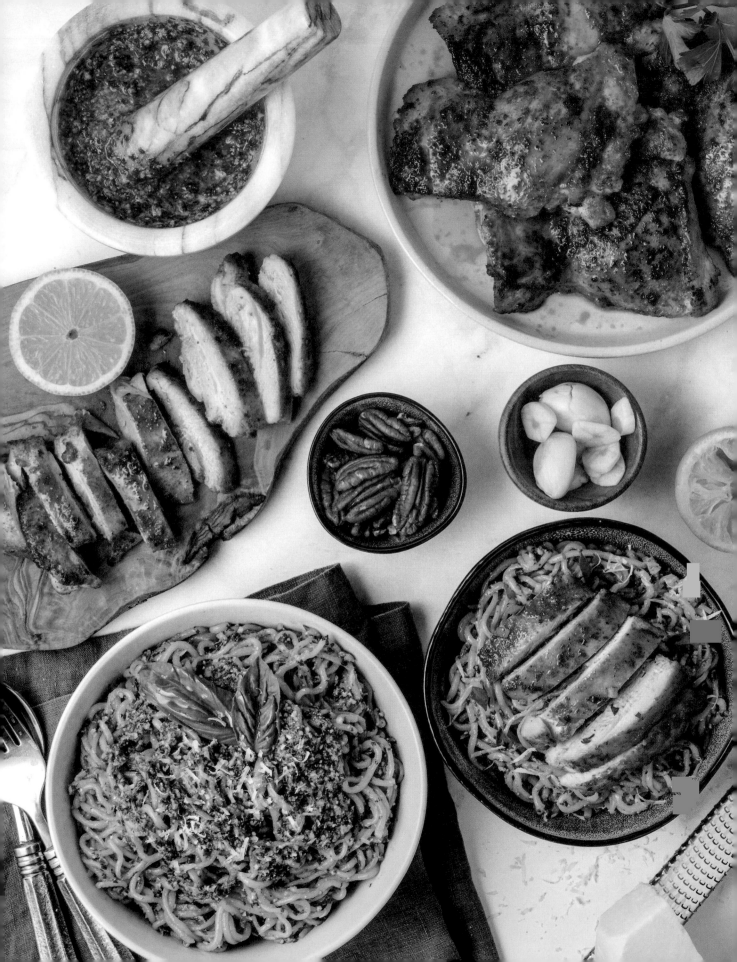

PREP TIME: **10 MINUTES** • COOKING TIME: **20 MINUTES** • MAKES: **5 MEALS**

PESTO PASTA
WITH SPICE-CRUSTED CHICKEN

I'll bet you thought eating a big bowl of pasta was off limits for keto? I did too, until I found the wonder know as shirataki noodles! Toss in a fresh pesto sauce and top with Italian spice-crusted chicken thighs for the ultimate bowl of keto pasta.

Tip You can buy "pasta zero by Nasoya" shirataki noodles at Whole Foods and Walmart. They have no odor and are a fantastic low-carb, low-calorie noodle option.

To watch the video tutorial for this recipe, search "FlavCity master class" on YouTube.

FOR THE CHICKEN:

- 1 teaspoon sweet paprika
- 1 teaspoon garlic powder
- 1 teaspoon onion powder
- ½ teaspoon dried oregano
- ¼ teaspoon cayenne pepper
- 10 boneless and skinless chicken thighs
- Kosher salt and fresh pepper
- Olive or avocado oil

FOR THE PESTO PASTA:

- 5 bags of shirataki noodles, 8 ounces each
- 1 cup Italian flat leaf parsley
- 1 cup fresh basil
- 2 cloves of garlic
- Zest of ½ lemon and 1 tablespoon of lemon juice
- ⅓ cup pecans, roasted if desired
- ¼ cup fresh grated Parmesan or Pecorino Romano cheese
- ¼ cup extra virgin olive oil
- ¼ teaspoon kosher salt
- Couple cracks fresh pepper

Make the spice rub by combining the paprika, onion and garlic powder, oregano, and cayenne pepper in a small bowl, and mix well. Season the chicken thighs with a generous pinch of salt and spice rub on each side. Rub the spice rub all around the chicken and allow to sit at room temperature for 15–20 minutes. Preheat a large pan, preferably cast-iron, over medium-high heat for 2 minutes. Add 2 teaspoons of oil, wait 30 seconds, then add the chicken. Cook 4 minutes without touching the chicken, flip and cook another 4 minutes. Set aside. You will have to work in two batches as to not overcrowd the pan.

For the pasta, drain the shirataki noodles well and place in a non-stick pan. Cook over medium heat for 8 minutes so excess moisture can evaporate. You know the noodles are ready when the bottom of the pan is white and dry. Remove noodles from pan, roughly chop them a couple times, and set aside.

Make the pesto by adding the parsley, basil, garlic, lemon zest and juice, pecans, salt, and pepper to a food processor and blend until everything is well combined, about 10–15 seconds. With the machine running, slowly add the olive oil and process until combined and very smooth. Add the cheese and process another 10 seconds. Turn the machine off and taste the pesto since it might need more cheese or lemon juice. If the consistency is a little dry, add 2–4 tablespoons more oil while the machine is running.

Add the noodles to a clean bowl and add enough pesto to coat and toss well, adding more pesto if needed. Serve pasta and top with sliced chicken.

STORAGE AND REHEATING: Save any leftover pesto in the fridge for five days. Pasta and chicken will keep in the fridge for five days. The chicken can be frozen, but the noodles can't. The best way to reheat is in a hot non-stick pan. If using the microwave, place a wet paper towel over the container and make sure not to overheat or the food will dry out.

MACROS

per meal with 2 chicken thighs (makes 5):
528 calories
2.9 grams of net carbs
8.8 grams of total carbs
27.2 grams of fat
24.2 grams of protein
7 grams of fiber

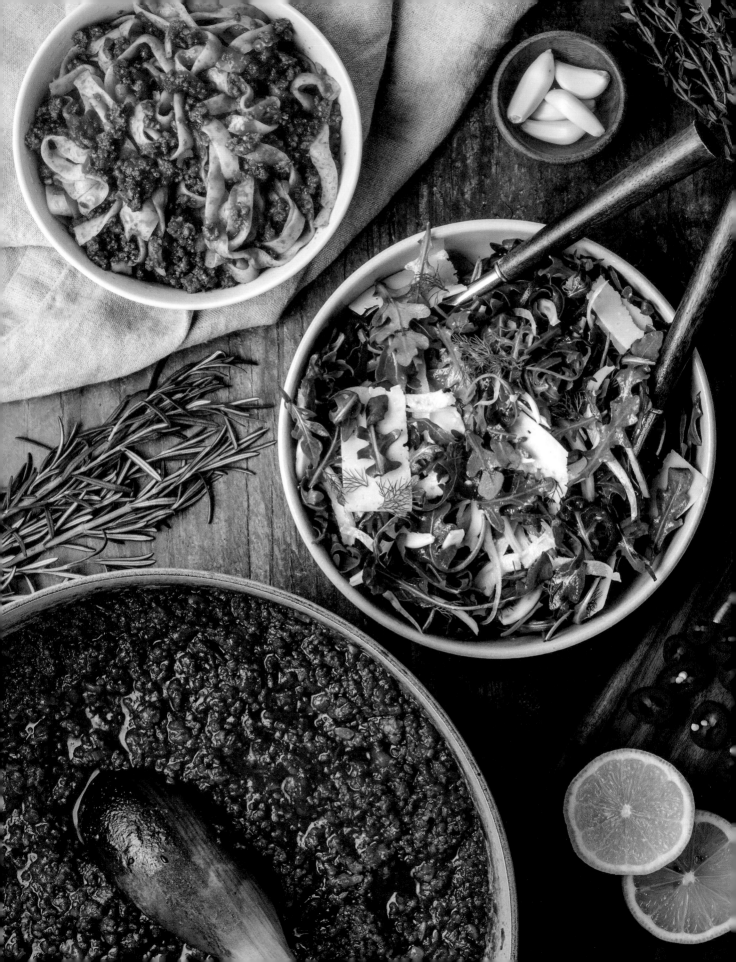

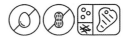

PREP TIME: **20 MINUTES** • COOKING TIME: **2 HOURS** • MAKES: **5 MEALS**

FETTUCCINE BOLOGNESE
WITH ARUGULA SALAD

If you thought the days of slurping down a big bowl of pasta and sauce were over just because you're on keto, think again my friends! This ragù Bolognese is so good that you could pour it over a shoe, and it would taste good. Mangia!

To watch a similar video tutorial for this recipe, search "FlavCity healthy spaghetti" on YouTube.

FOR THE PASTA AND RAGÙ:

- 1 yellow onion, finely chopped
- 2 stalks celery, chopped
- 2 teaspoons fresh thyme, finely chopped
- 2 teaspoons rosemary, finely chopped
- ½ teaspoon red pepper flakes
- 4 cloves garlic, minced
- 2 heaping tablespoons tomato paste
- ⅔ pound ground veal
- ⅔ pound ground beef
- ⅔ pound ground pork
- ½ cup red wine, like pinot or cabernet
- 1 twenty-eight-ounce can whole Italian San Marzano tomatoes
- 1 bay leaf
- 5 bags of shirataki fettuccine noodles, 8 ounces each
- Freshly chopped parsley
- Kosher salt and fresh pepper
- Olive oil
- Pecorino Romano or Parmesan cheese

FOR THE SALAD:

- 12–14 ounces of arugula
- 1 fennel bulb, thinly sliced
- 1–2 long, thin red chili peppers, sliced
- Shaved Pecorino or Parmesan cheese
- 2 lemons
- Extra virgin olive oil
- Kosher salt and fresh pepper

Start the ragù by preheating a tall-sided pan or Dutch oven just above medium heat along with 2 tablespoons of oil. Add the onion, celery, thyme, rosemary, red pepper flakes, ½ teaspoon salt, and a few cracks of pepper. Mix well and cook for 15–20 minutes or until the veggies are very soft and have wilted down. Add one more tablespoon of oil, as well as the garlic and tomato paste, and cook for 3 minutes. Raise the heat to medium-high and add the veal, beef, and pork, along with ½ teaspoon salt, and a few cracks of pepper. Cook until the ground meats have just cooked through; use a spatula to break them up. Then add the red wine, mix well, and cook until almost all the wine has reduced. Crush the canned tomatoes using your hands or use a potato masher and add them to the pot. Add ½ cup of water to the tomato tin to remove any leftovers and add that to the pan along with the bay leaf, ¾ teaspoon salt and a few cracks of black pepper. Stir well and bring to simmer. Reduce to a very low simmer and allow to cook with the lid on for 2 hours. Stir every 30 minutes and add more water if the ragù gets too thick. Check for seasoning halfway, you may need more salt. After 2 hours, remove the lid and keep cooking until the ragù has thickened to a proper consistency. Set aside.

Drain the shirataki noodles thoroughly and cook them in a non-stick pan over medium-high heat for 8 minutes. This will remove the excess moisture. You'll know the noodles are ready when the bottom of the pan is coated in a dry white residue. Take off the heat and set aside. Use a knife or scissors to cut the noodles a few times, otherwise they tend to clump together in one giant ball.

Add as much ragù as needed to the pan with the noodles and cook over medium heat for 3 minutes, so the sauce can really coat the noodles. Turn the heat off, add parsley, and mix well.

Make the salad by adding the arugula to a large bowl. Use a hand slicer or a knife to thinly slice the fennel, and then roughly chop it with a knife. Add the fennel to the arugula along with the shaved cheese (use a veggie peeler), and sliced chilies. Store the salad in an air tight container in the fridge. When ready to eat, dress each portion with a drizzle of oil, some lemon juice, a tiny pinch of salt, and a crack of pepper. Toss and enjoy. Only dress the salad right before you want to eat it, otherwise it will get soggy.

Before digging in, grate a generous amount of cheese over the bowl of pasta and add a drizzle of good extra virgin olive oil if you have it. Enjoy!

STORAGE AND REHEATING: The pasta and meat sauce will keep in the fridge for five days; the ragù can be frozen for two to three months, but not the noodles. The undressed salad will keep in the fridge for five days but can't be frozen. The best way to reheat the pasta is in a hot non-stick pan. Otherwise, take the lid off the container, cover with tin foil, and reheat in a 350°F oven for 10 minutes. If reheating in the microwave, take the lid off and cover with a wet paper towel. Make sure not to reheat too long or the ragù will dry out.

MACROS

per serving of pasta (makes 5):
473 calories
9.9 grams of net carbs
20.3 grams of total carbs
28.6 grams of fat
36.4 grams of protein
8.7 grams of fiber

MACROS

per serving of salad (makes 5):
97 calories
2.4 grams of net carbs
4.6 grams of total carbs
7.6 grams of fat
4.3 grams of protein
2.2 grams of fiber

★★★★★

"I made this and was so impressed! I was really concerned about the noodles. But after rinsing them well and cooking out the water on the stovetop, they just absorbed all the deliciousness of the sauce. Cooking out the water on the stovetop is such a brilliant idea! Thank you! I've been loving this lunch all week!" —**Pineapple**

"Bought those noodles today and made spaghetti. Thank you for showing us ways to eat well but healthy." —**Angelia S.**

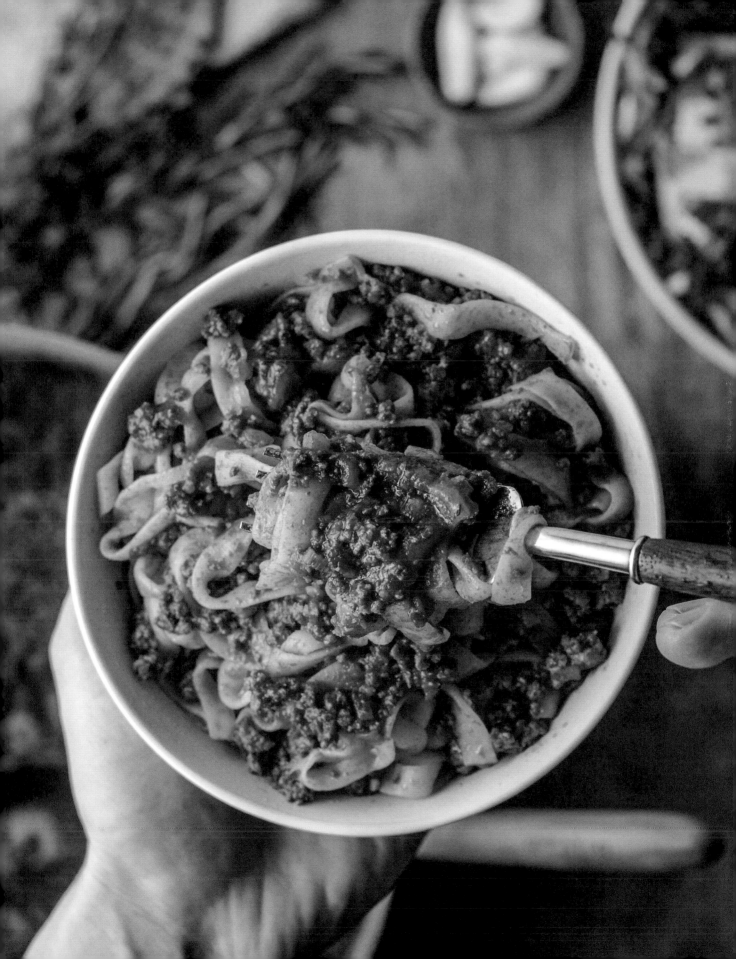

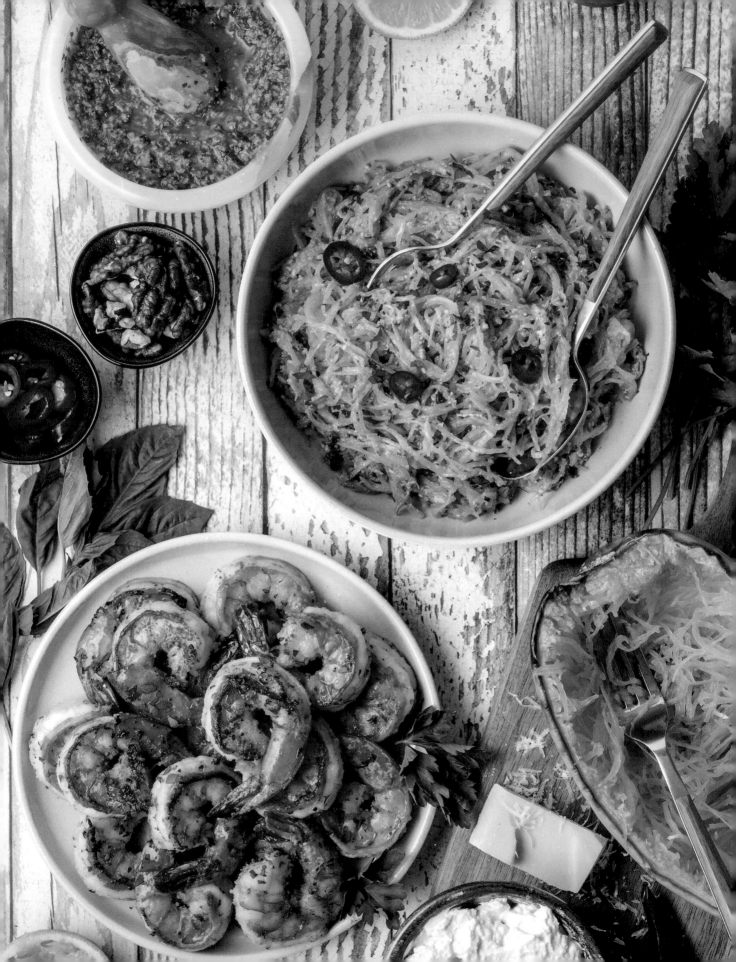

PREP TIME: **15 MINUTES** • COOKING TIME: **60 MINUTES** • MAKES: **5 MEALS**

SPAGHETTI SQUASH PESTO
WITH SHRIMP

This recipe is what I call a culinary fake-out. I love the way spaghetti squash pulls into long strands after it's roasted. Once you toss it with creamy ricotta pesto and top it with juicy shrimp, your pasta craving will be satisfied.

To watch the video tutorial for this recipe, search "FlavCity spaghetti squash pesto" on YouTube.

FOR THE SQUASH:

- 7½ cups of cooked spaghetti squash, about 5½ pound raw squash
- Zest and juice of ½ lemon
- 1 long thin red-hot chili pepper or pepper flakes
- Olive oil
- Kosher salt and fresh pepper

FOR THE PESTO:

- ¼ cup roasted and unsalted walnuts
- 1 cup Italian flat leaf parsley
- 1 cup pack fresh basil
- 2 cloves of garlic
- Zest and juice of ½ lemon
- ¼ cup grated Pecorino Romano or Parmesan cheese
- ¼ cup whole milk ricotta cheese
- ¼ cup extra virgin olive oil
- Kosher salt and fresh pepper

FOR THE SHRIMP:

- 2 pounds of raw, shelled, and cleaned shrimp
- 1 teaspoon onion powder
- 1 teaspoon garlic powder
- 1 teaspoon dried oregano
- Olive oil
- Kosher salt and fresh pepper

For the squash, preheat oven to 400°F. Carefully cut the squash in half from top to bottom using a knife and a rolling pin. Scoop out the seeds and save them for roasting and snacking while watching Netflix. Roast on a sheet tray, cut side up, for 60–75 minutes or until the flesh can easily be pierced with a knife. Set aside, so the squash can cool a bit.

While the squash is cooking, **make the pesto** by adding the walnuts to a food processor and pulse for 10 seconds. Add ¼ teaspoon of salt, a few cracks of pepper, and the remaining ingredients except the ricotta, Pecorino, and olive oil, and run the processor until everything is well combined, about 10–15 seconds. With the machine running, slowly add olive oil until the mixture is smooth, loose, and creamy. Add the ricotta and Pecorino cheese and process another 10 seconds. Turn the machine off and taste the pesto; it might need more cheese or lemon juice. If the consistency is dry, add more oil while the machine is running. Set aside.

Once the squash has cooled a bit, use a fork to rake the surface from top to bottom. Place all the spaghetti strands in a large bowl and add the lemon zest and juice along with ½ teaspoon of salt. Add enough pesto to thoroughly coat the squash and mix well. Finely slice the chili pepper and add that to the spaghetti, or add a pinch of red pepper flakes. Check for seasoning, you will likely need a squeeze of lemon juice and maybe a pinch of salt. Set aside.

Make the shrimp. Be sure the shrimp are very dry, otherwise pat them dry with paper towels, and season with 1 teaspoon oil, the onion and garlic powder, oregano, ¾ teaspoon salt, and a few cracks of pepper, and mix well. Preheat a large cast-iron pan over medium-high heat for 2 minutes with 1 tablespoon of oil. Add half the shrimp to the pan and cook for 2 minutes on the first side; flip, and only cook 1–2 minutes on the second side. Remove shrimp from pan, add more oil, and cook the second batch.

Serve the spaghetti squash pesto with the shrimp and enjoy!

STORAGE AND REHEATING: The squash pesto will last in the fridge for five days but can't be frozen, and the shrimp will last for three days in the fridge. Make more shrimp on day three or freeze some, although I don't like frozen shrimp; they get rubbery. The best way to reheat the squash pesto and shrimp is in a hot non-stick pan for a few minutes; otherwise cover the container with a wet paper towel and gently reheat in the microwave, making sure not to overcook the shrimp.

MACROS

per serving of squash and shrimp (makes 5):

475 calories

15.4 grams of net carbs

19.2 grams of total carbs

26.9 grams of fat

3.75 grams of protein

3.7 grams of fiber

★★★★★

"Omg!! I made this last night. It was the bomb.com!!" —**Sharon H.**

PREP TIME: **20 MINUTES** • COOKING TIME: **30 MINUTES** • MAKES: **5 MEALS**

BEEF LETTUCE WRAPS
WITH SESAME NOODLE SALAD

This is a healthy version of your favorite P.F. Chang's menu item. The beef wraps are juicy and crispy, and the flavors just pop in your mouth. The noodle salad is meant to be eaten cold and has lots of crunchy veggies along with a dynamite almond butter dressing.

 Tip | My favorite brand of shirataki noodles is called "Pasta zero by Nasoya." They don't have a weird smell or funky texture, and you can buy them at Whole Foods or Walmart.

 | To watch the video tutorial for this recipe, search "FlavCity lettuce wraps" on YouTube.

FOR THE BEEF LETTUCE WRAPS:
- ½ onion, chopped
- 2 pounds ground beef, 80:20 beef to fat ratio
- 3 cloves garlic, minced
- 1 teaspoon fresh ginger, finely grated
- 2 teaspoons sambal oelek chili paste or sriracha
- 3 tablespoons tamari soy sauce
- 1 teaspoon toasted sesame oil
- Lime juice
- 2–3 tablespoons unsalted and roasted peanuts, chopped
- 3 tablespoons green onions, finely sliced
- 2 heads of butter lettuce or romaine lettuce
- 2 red-hot chili peppers, thinly sliced for garnish
- Avocado or coconut oil
- Kosher salt and fresh pepper

FOR THE NOODLE SALAD:
- ½ cup smooth almond butter
- 2 tablespoons tamari soy sauce
- 1–2 teaspoons sambal oelek chili paste or sriracha
- 1 clove garlic
- Juice of ½ lime
- 3 drops of liquid stevia
- 1 teaspoon toasted sesame oil
- Cold water
- 2 pounds of shirataki noodles
- ½ red bell pepper, thinly sliced
- 1 cup snow peas, thinly sliced on the angle
- 2 tablespoons green onions, finely sliced
- 2 tablespoons fresh mint, chopped
- 1 teaspoon sesame seeds, toasted if desired

For the lettuce wraps, preheat a large non-stick pan over medium-high heat for 2 minutes along with 1 tablespoon of oil. Add the onions, ¼ teaspoon salt, a couple cracks of pepper, and cook for 3 minutes. Add the beef, along with ¼ teaspoon salt, and use a spatula to break the beef into small pieces. Cook for 3 minutes and then add the garlic and ginger. Continue cooking a few more minutes until most of the pink color is gone from the beef and lower the heat to low. Add the chili paste, tamari, sesame oil, and a little squeeze of lime; mix well. Turn the heat off as soon as the ground beef is cooked through. Otherwise the beef will dry out. Check for seasoning; you will most likely need more tamari or chili paste, depending on your preference. Add the peanuts and green onions, mix well and set aside.

For the almond dressing, add the almond butter to a food processor, blender, or use a bowl with a whisk. Add the tamari, sambal oelek, garlic, lime juice, stevia, sesame oil, and ¼ cup of cold water. Blend until the sauce is creamy and pourable, adding more water as needed. Check for seasoning, you will definitely need to adjust based upon your preference of heat, salt, sweet, or vinegar.

Drain the shirataki noodles thoroughly and cook them in a non-stick pan over high heat for 6–8 minutes. This will remove the excess moisture. You'll know the noodles are ready when the bottom of the pan is coated in a dry white residue. Take off the heat, roughly chop, and add them to a large bowl. Season them with the juice of half a lime and 1 tablespoon of tamari. Add enough almond dressing to thoroughly coat the noodles and toss well. Add the sliced red bell peppers, snow peas, green onions, mint, and sesame seeds, and mix well.

To assemble the beef wraps, place a scoop of the beef mixture in a piece of lettuce, and garnish with sliced red chilies and green onions. Serve with some noodle salad and enjoy!

STORAGE AND REHEATING: Store the beef mixture separately from the noodle salad. Each will keep in the fridge for five days. The beef mixture can be frozen for two to three months. The noodles can't be frozen. Reheat beef in a 350°F oven for 10 minutes. If reheating in the microwave, take the lid off, cover with a wet paper towel, and make sure not to reheat too long or the beef will dry out. Don't heat the noodle salad.

MACROS

per serving wraps (makes 5):
521 calories
2.5 grams of net carbs
3.3 grams of net carbs
39.5 grams of fat
32.9 grams of protein
0.7 grams of fiber

MACROS

per serving of noodles (makes 5):
219 calories
6.9 grams of net carbs
15 grams of total carbs
15.5 grams of fat
7.9 grams of protein
8.3 grams of fiber

★★★★★

"I love love love this recipe. Soooo damn tasty. Family favorite once again!" —**Saniahmylove**

"This is, hands down, the tastiest thing that has ever been made in my kitchen. And I cook A LOT. I couldn't find the noodles at Whole Foods or TJs, and I wasn't interested in extending my search, so I spiralized carrots and uses carrot "noodles." That seemed, to me, to be the perfect sub. SO good. I made this Sunday afternoon and went to bed excited for my lunch break today!" —**Danielle M.**

"Made this for dinner tonight and it was delicious! The meat is sooo flavorful and has just the right balance of spice. I love it and I love your videos! Thanks for the recipe, keep 'em coming!" —**Katie B.**

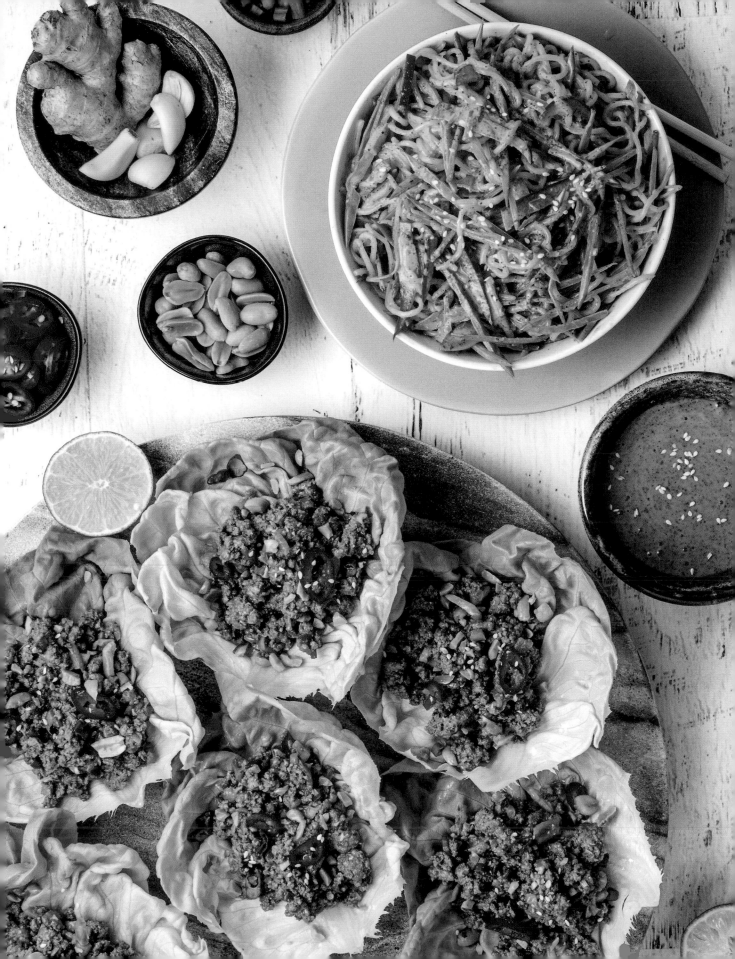

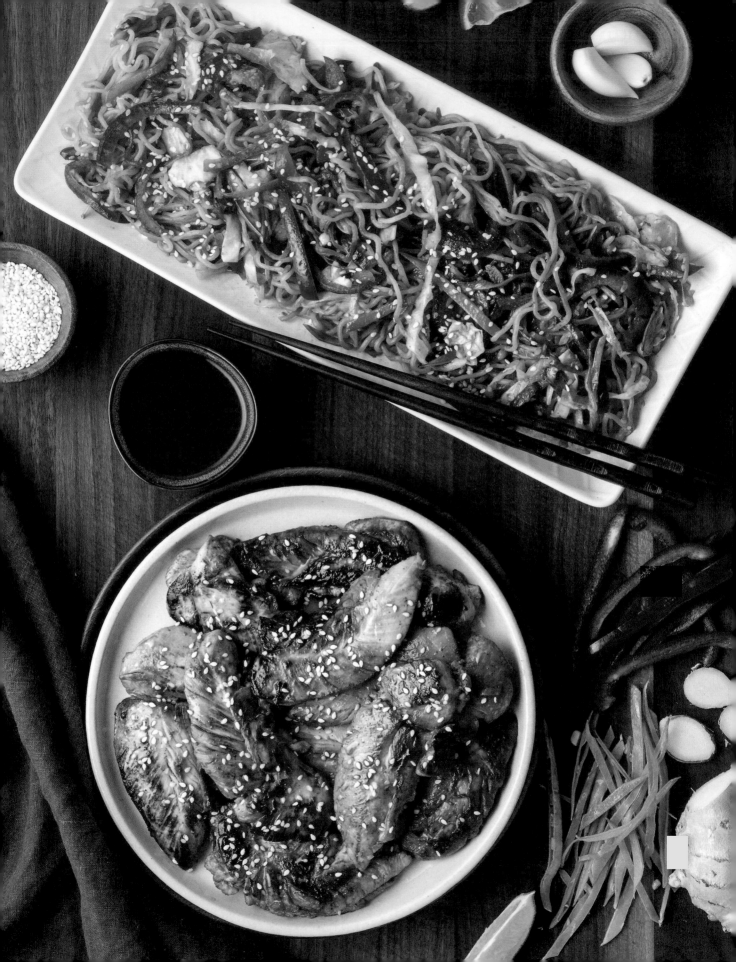

PREP TIME: **20 MINUTES** • COOKING TIME: **70 MINUTES** • MAKES: **5 MEALS**

SESAME CHICKEN
AND VEGGIE STIR-FRY

I love recipes that use the same ingredients more than once, so I decided to do it three times! The Asian marinade also doubles as the stir-fry sauce, and, once simmered and reduced, it's the sauce that gets poured over the juicy marinated chicken.

Tip | You can buy chicken breasts and cut them yourself, or buy breasts and ask the butcher in the grocery store to do it for you. Each breast should make three or four strips, roughly one inch wide.

Tip | I prefer to use sambal oelek chili paste (rooster on bottle) instead of sriracha. It has no sugar or carbs.

FOR THE CHICKEN:

- ½ cup tamari soy sauce
- Juice of ½ lime
- 1½ teaspoons toasted sesame oil
- 1–2 tablespoon sambal oelek or chili sauce
- 6 drops liquid stevia
- 2 pounds boneless and skinless chicken breast strips
- ½ teaspoon sesame seeds
- Avocado oil

FOR THE VEGGIE STIR-FRY:

- 2 pounds of shirataki noodles
- 2 teaspoons sambal oelek or sriracha
- 3 tablespoons tamari soy sauce or coconut aminos
- 1 teaspoon toasted sesame seed oil
- Juice of ½ lime
- 1 red pepper, thinly sliced
- ½ red onion, sliced
- 1 cup snow peas, thinly sliced on an angle
- 3 cloves garlic, minced
- 1 teaspoon fresh ginger, finely grated
- 1 cup green cabbage, finely sliced
- 1 teaspoon sesame seeds
- Avocado oil

Make the marinade for the chicken by combining the tamari, sesame oil, sambal, lime juice, and stevia in a small bowl. Mix well and give it a taste. You want a good balance of flavors, so add more of whatever you feel is lacking. Place the chicken strips in a tight-fitting dish or bowl and pour the marinade over. Press the chicken down with your hands and let marinate at room temperature while you cook the veggies and noodles.

To make the stir-fry, thoroughly drain the shirataki noodles from the water in the package and preheat a large non-stick pan over medium-high heat for 1 minute. Add the noodles to the pan and cook for 7 minutes, stirring often so the excess water in the noodles can evaporate. If you skip this step, the stir-fry will be very watery. Meanwhile, make the stir-fry sauce by adding the sambal, tamari, sesame oil, and lime juice to a small bowl. Mix well and set aside. Remove noodles, roughly chop them, and set side. Add 2 teaspoons of oil to the same pan over medium-high heat along with the red peppers, snow peas, and red onions. Cook for 5 minutes, stirring often or until the veggies have softened a little bit. Add the garlic and ginger and cook for 2 minutes. Add the cabbage and noodles to the pan along with the stir-fry sauce. Mix well and cook for 2 minutes. Check the noodles for seasoning as you may need to mix up more stir-fry sauce. Turn the heat off, add the sesame seeds, mix well, and set aside.

To cook the chicken, remove it from the marinade and thoroughly pat dry with paper towels. Pour the leftover marinade in a small pot and set aside. Preheat a large pan over medium-high heat with 1 tablespoon of oil for 2 minutes. Add half of the chicken to the pan and cook for 4 minutes. Once the bottom of the chicken has some dark color, flip and cook another 4 minutes. Remove from the pan, add a little more oil, and cook the second batch of chicken.

While the chicken is cooking, bring the leftover marinade to a boil for 1 minute and then reduce to a simmer. Cook until reduced and has a saucy consistency. Pour the sauce all over the cooked chicken and garnish with ½ teaspoon of sesame seeds. Enjoy!

Keto Meal Prep

STORAGE AND REHEATING: Everything will keep in the fridge for five days. You can freeze the chicken for two to three months but not the noodles. Reheat in a 350°F oven for 7–10 minutes. If reheating in the microwave, take the lid off, cover with a wet paper towel, and make sure not to reheat too long or the chicken will dry out.

MACROS

per serving of chicken (makes 5):
271 calories
1.5 grams of net and total carbs
8.9 grams of fat
58 grams of protein
0.2 grams of fiber

MACROS

per serving of noodles (makes 5):
76 calories
6.1 grams of net carbs
12.1 grams of total carbs
3.1 grams of fat
2 grams of protein
6.7 grams of fiber

★★★★★

"Hey Bobby, I just made this. Oh boy! One for my belly for lunch, four more for next week. Thanks, keep the vids coming." —**John B.**

"I just made this and OMG it is delicious! Thanks Bobby you have yourself a new happy subscriber!" —**Marlee**

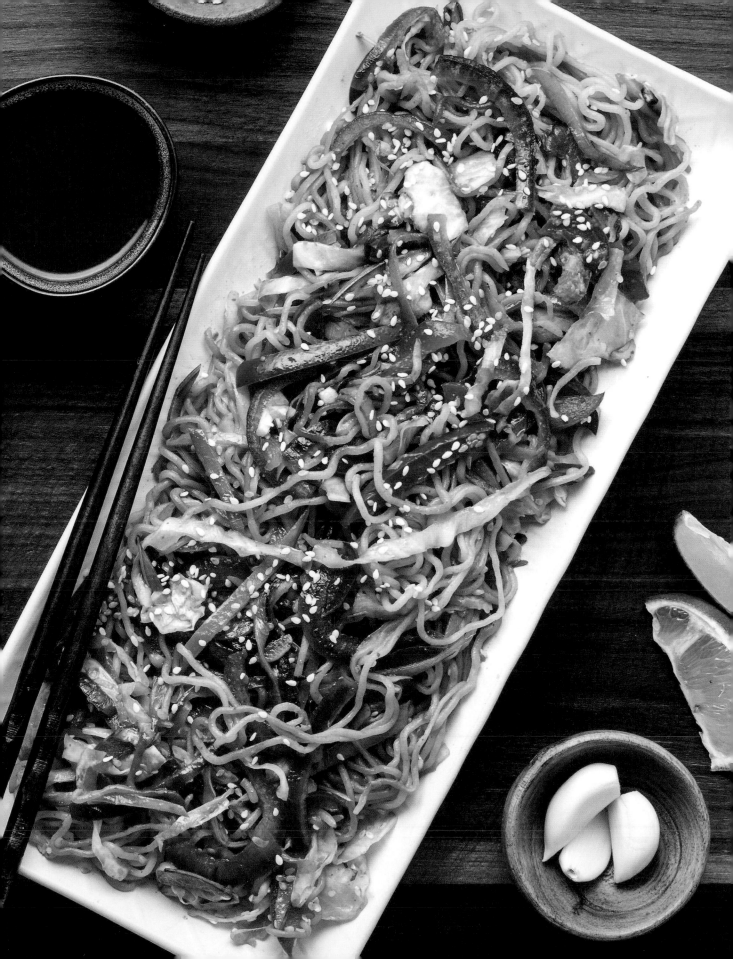

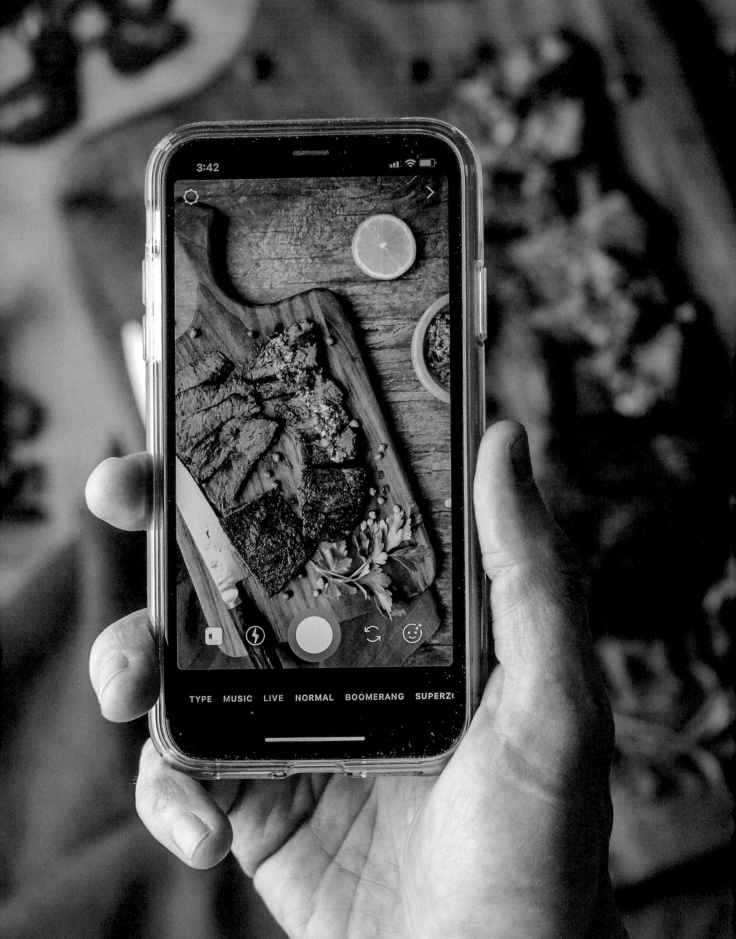

BEEF—RAISING THE STEAKS

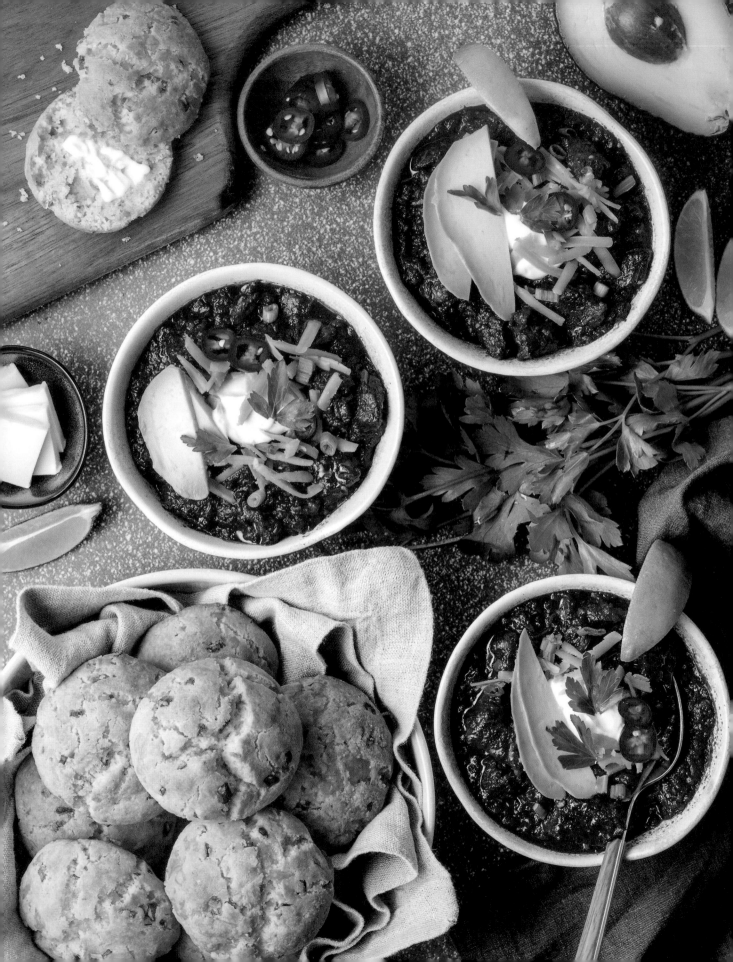

PREP TIME: **30 MINUTES** • COOKING TIME: **2 HOURS** • MAKES: **5 MEALS**

BEEF CHILI
AND CHEDDAR BISCUITS

If you want to step up your next Netflix and chill night, then you need to make this recipe. The chili is loaded with flavor and everything you crave on a cold day. These biscuits are my take on Red Lobster's buttery biscuits. It's hard to believe they are grain free and keto!

Tip | If using a slow cooker, first cook the onions and bacon in a cast-iron pan, then use then same pan to brown the beef. Follow the rest of the instructions and cook for 6–8 hours in your slow cooker.

| To watch the video tutorial for this recipe, search "FlavCity chili" on YouTube.

FOR THE CHILI:

- 3 dried ancho or chipotle chilies, seeds removed
- 3 cloves of garlic, peeled
- 1½ teaspoons ancho chili powder
- 1½ teaspoons smoked paprika
- 1½ teaspoons cumin
- 1 teaspoon dried oregano
- Heaping ¼ teaspoon cinnamon
- 3 small tomatillos
- 1 poblano pepper
- 4 ounces sugar-free bacon, cubed
- 1 cup chopped onions
- 2 pounds of beef stew meat or brisket, cut in one-inch cubes
- 20 ounces of canned crushed tomatoes
- Olive or avocado oil
- Stevia drops, optional
- Kosher salt and fresh pepper

FOR THE BISCUITS:

- See recipe on page 159

For the chili, soak the dry ancho or chipotle chilies in just boiled water for at least 20 minutes. Transfer chilies to a blender with 1 cup of the soaking liquid along with the garlic, ancho chili powder, smoked paprika, cumin, oregano, and cinnamon. Blend well and set aside.

Preheat the broiler to high and peel the outer paper off the tomatillos and place them on a sheet tray with the poblano pepper. Broil for about 10 minutes or until evenly charred on all sides, making sure to turn the poblano and tomatillos. Once the pepper has cooled down, run some cold water over it and remove the seeds and try to peel away most of the charred skin. Add the poblano and tomatillos to the blender with the chili mixture and blend until smooth.

Preheat a large stock pot or Dutch oven over medium heat along with 2 teaspoons of oil. Add the bacon and cook until most of the fat has rendered off—about 8–10 minutes. Add the onions and cook until they are very soft—about 10–12 minutes. Use a spoon and transfer onions and bacon to a bowl. Raise the heat to just below high and add 1 tablespoon of oil. Season the beef stew meat with a generous amount of salt and pepper and sear until brown on all sides—about 7–8 minutes. Turn the heat down to medium. Add the bacon, onion, and blended chili mixture to the pot along with the canned tomatoes. Add enough water to cover everything by 3 inches and bring the chili to a simmer. Place a lid on the pot and cook for 2 hours, stirring a few times. After 30 minutes, check for seasoning. If the chili gets too thick, just add more water. After 2 hours, take the lid off and see if the chili needs a few drops of stevia to balance the heat and acid from the tomatoes. Use a large spoon or spatula to mash to beef cubes into small pieces—this will help make the chili thicker. Remove the heat from the chili and set aside. Chili will get better the next day.

While the chili is cooking, **make the biscuits** by following the instructions on page 159.

Serve the chili with the biscuits and your favorite toppings and enjoy!

STORAGE AND REHEATING: Chili will keep in the fridge for five days or can be frozen for two to three months. Biscuits will keep in the fridge for three to four days or can be frozen for two to three months.

MACROS

per serving of chili (makes 5):
506 calories
6.5 grams of net carbs
8.1 grams of total carbs
25.6 grams of fat
44 grams of protein
1.5 grams of fiber

MACROS

per biscuit (makes 10):
230 calories
1.8 net grams of carbs
3.6 grams of total carbs
22.4 grams of fat
6.2 grams of protein
1.8 grams of fiber

★★★★★

"I made this last night in the crockpot. Everyone at work said my lunch smelled the best. I was not sharing. Another successful recipe. Thanks Bobby! My go-to chili recipe!" —**Bekie B**

"Best chili I've ever made!!!" —**Scott C.**

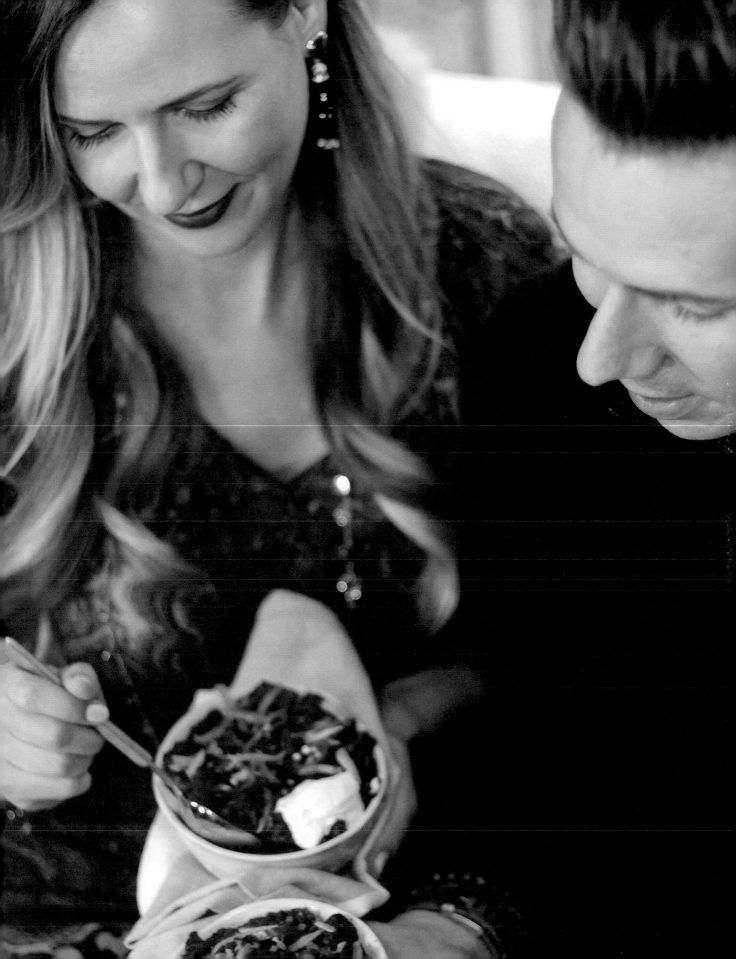

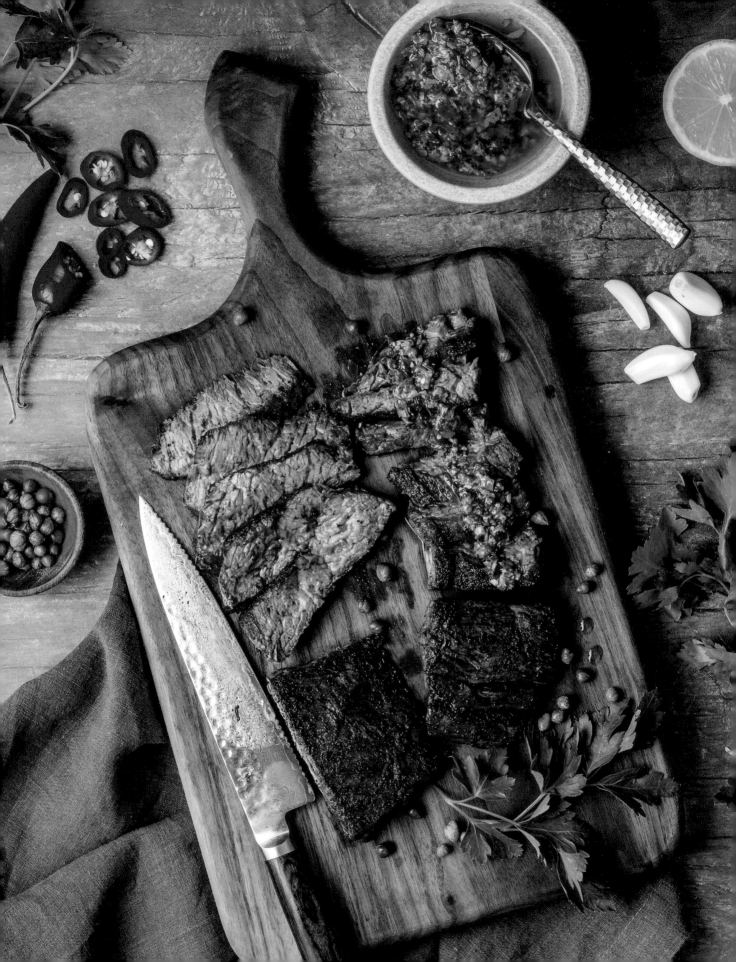

PREP TIME: **5 MINUTES** • COOKING TIME: **10 MINUTES** • MAKES: **2 SERVINGS**

PALEO

COFFEE-RUBBED SKIRT STEAK
WITH SALSA VERDE

You know the secret spice rubs that BBQ pit masters use for ribs and pulled pork? This is my version of that. The only difference is that I will tell you my recipe. Good luck getting it from those folks! The coffee rub has insane flavors. Feel free to use on chicken, pork, or other cuts of beef. Same goes for the salsa verde—it's the perfect condiment for cutting through a rich and fatty piece of meat.

 To watch the video tutorial for this recipe, search "FlavCity steak four ways" on YouTube.

FOR THE SPICE RUB:

- 1 ¼ tablespoons finely ground coffee
- 1 tablespoon ancho chili powder
- ½ tablespoon smoked paprika
- ½ tablespoon ground cumin
- ½ teaspoon ground cinnamon
- ½ teaspoon ground coriander
- 1 tablespoon brown sugar substitute, like Sukrin Gold
- 1 teaspoon dried thyme
- ½ teaspoon cayenne pepper

FOR THE STEAK:

- 2–4 skirt steaks, 5–8 ounces each
- Kosher salt
- Avocado oil

FOR THE SALSA VERDE:

- ¼ cup extra virgin olive oil
- 2 teaspoons freshly chopped parsley
- Zest and juice of ½ lemon
- 1 teaspoon capers, drained and finely minced
- 1 clove garlic, grated
- 1 teaspoon Dijon or stone-ground mustard
- ½ red chili, minced or ¼ teaspoon red pepper flakes
- Pinch of salt and two cracks of black pepper

To make the spice rub, combine all ingredients in a small bowl and mix well. Add a generous pinch of salt and spice rub to the skirt steak and allow to sit at room temperature for 20–30 minutes. Store leftover spice rub in an air tight container for three to six months. Never add salt to the spice rubs. Salt should be added separately to the meat when you season it.

Make the salsa verde by combing all the ingredients in a bowl and mix well. Check for seasoning; you want the flavors to be bold, so adjust accordingly.

To cook the steak, preheat a cast-iron pan over medium-high heat for 3 minutes. Add 1 tablespoon of oil, wait for it to heat up. Add the steaks and push down for 5 seconds so they make good contact with the pan. Cook for 3 minutes or until nice and crusty and flip. Cook another 3 minutes and remove from pan. If you like skirt steak cooked medium, cook an additional 1 minute per side.

Allow the steak to rest under aluminum foil for 5 minutes so the juices can redistribute. Cut the steak in half a couple times and then slice it against the grain. This will ensure the meat melts in your mouth. Never cut skirt steak with the grain. Spoon over some salsa verde and enjoy.

STORAGE AND REHEATING: Steak and salsa will keep in the fridge for four to five days and should be reheated in a 350°F oven for 7–10 minutes with the salsa spooned over the top so that the meat does not dry out. Both items can be frozen for two to three months.

MACROS

per skirt steak:
512 calories
Less than 1 gram net and total carbs
34 grams of fat
42 grams of protein
0 fiber

MACROS

for all the salsa verde:
501 calories
0.89 grams of net carbs
1 total grams of carbs
56 grams of fat
0 protein
0 fiber

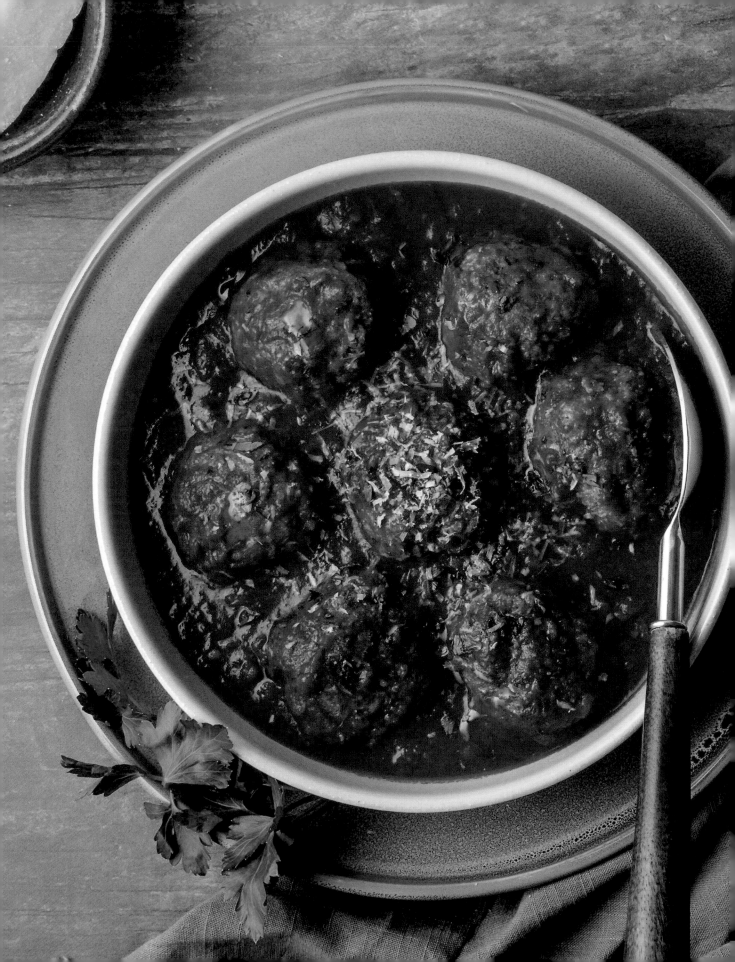

PREP TIME: **20 MINUTES** • COOKING TIME: **1 HOUR** • MAKES: **13 MEATBALLS**

NONNA'S
MEATBALLS AND SAUCE

In my mind, Nonna was from the Amalfi Coast and taught me this recipe while cooking in her lemon orchard. In reality, my Jewish bubble *was from the northside of Chicago, and it just so happens that she really loved my meatball recipe. That still counts for something!*

Tip | **Want to save yourself some time? Instead of making my homemade sauce, buy Rao's marinara. It's my favorite brand and Costco has the best price.**

FOR THE MARINARA SAUCE:

- 1 medium-sized onion, chopped
- 1 large zucchini chopped
- 2 stalks celery, chopped
- ½ teaspoon dried thyme
- ¼ teaspoon red pepper flakes
- 4 cloves of garlic, finely diced
- 3 tablespoons tomato paste
- ½ cup red wine, like pinot noir
- 1 twenty-eight-ounce can whole San Marzano tomatoes
- Kosher salt and fresh pepper
- Olive oil

FOR THE MEATBALLS:

- ¾ cup almond flour
- ½ cup heavy cream or water
- ½ pound ground beef
- ½ pound ground pork
- ½ pound ground veal
- 1 heaping teaspoon onion powder
- 1 heaping teaspoon garlic powder
- 1 egg
- 1 tablespoon freshly chopped parsley
- ½ teaspoon dried oregano
- ¼ teaspoon red pepper flakes
- ¼ cup finely grated Pecorino Romano or Parmesan cheese
- Olive oil
- 1 teaspoon kosher salt
- Freshly cracked black pepper

For the marinara, preheat a large, heavy-bottom pot over medium heat with 2 tablespoons of oil. Add the onion, zucchini, celery, thyme, and pepper flakes, along with ½ teaspoon of salt and a couple cracks of pepper. Cook for 15 minutes or until the veggies are very soft and wilted. Add the garlic and cook for 5 minutes. Add the tomato paste and cook for 2 minutes. Then add the wine and sir well. Cook for 3 minutes until almost all the wine has reduced and then add the tomatoes (crushed by hand or potato masher) along with 1 cup of water. Season with ¾ teaspoon of salt and some pepper. Bring to a bare simmer and let cook uncovered for 45–60 minutes. If the sauce gets too thick, add more water. Check for seasoning halfway as you may need more salt. Turn the heat off the pot and set aside.

For the meatballs, add the almond flour to a bowl and cover with just enough cream to make it wet and mushy. To a separate large bowl, add the ground meats, onion and garlic powder, egg, parsley, oregano, pepper flakes, grated cheese, salt, and a few cracks of pepper. Add the almond flour mixture and mix with your hands until well combined, making sure not to overmix or the meatballs will be tough. Dip your hands in water and form meatballs; there should be enough for thirteen, but you can make them any size you desire.

Place meatballs in the fridge for 20 minutes to firm up, or you can store overnight. To sear the meatballs and make them crusty, preheat a non-stick pan over medium-high heat with 2 teaspoons of olive oil. Once the oil is hot, add half the meatballs and cook until crusty, about 1–2 minutes, and flip and repeat. You don't want to overcrowd the pan, so this needs to be done in two batches. Move the meatballs to the marinara sauce, bring to a gentle simmer, and cook for 30 minutes.

Plate the meatballs and sauce, and garnish with parsley, a drizzle of really good extra virgin olive oil, grated cheese, and enjoy!

STORAGE AND REHEATING: Meatballs can be stored with the sauce in the fridge for five days or everything can be frozen for three months. It's best to thaw the meatballs and sauce overnight before reheating in a pot over medium heat. If using a microwave, cover the container with a wet paper towel and make sure to not to overheat as the meatballs will get dry.

MACROS

per meatball (makes 13):
201 calories
1.2 grams of net carbs
2 grams of total carbs
6.2 grams of fat
12.3 grams of protein
0.8 grams of fiber

MACROS

for all the sauce (about 30 ounces):
536 calories
56 grams of net carbs
71 grams of total carbs
16 grams of fat
11.7 grams of protein
14.3 grams of fiber

PREP TIME: **20 MINUTES** • COOK TIME: **70 MINUTES** • MAKES: **5 MEALS**

CHEESY STUFFED MEATLOAF
WITH BROCCOLINI AND EGGPLANT

Not that meatloaf needed any help in the flavor department, but it can't hurt when it's stuffed with mozzarella cheese and prosciutto and baked in the oven. Served with a funky little side dish that has Japanese eggplant, broccolini, crispy garlic, and shallots. So good!

 Tip | Make homemade sugar-free ketchup by searching "FlavCity ketchup" on YouTube. It's a new recipe that did not make the book.

 You Tube | To watch the video tutorial for this recipe, search "FlavCity meatloaf" on YouTube.

FOR THE MEATLOAF:

- ½ red onion, diced
- 1 green bell pepper, diced
- ½ teaspoon dried thyme
- 3 cloves garlic, minced
- 2 pounds ground beef, 80:20 beef to fat ratio
- 2 eggs
- ¼ cup grated Parmesan or Pecorino Romano cheese
- 5 ounces sliced provolone cheese
- ¼ pound sliced prosciutto, optional
- Keto ketchup, no sugar added
- Kosher salt and fresh pepper
- Avocado or olive oil

FOR THE VEGGIES:

- 1 pound broccolini or baby broccoli
- 1 large Japanese eggplant
- 1 large shallot, thinly sliced
- 3 cloves garlic, thinly sliced
- 1 teaspoon mustard seeds
- Zest and juice of ½ lemon
- Kosher salt and fresh pepper
- Avocado or olive oil

For the meatloaf, preheat oven to 350°F. Preheat a large non-stick pan over medium heat along with 1 tablespoon of oil. Add the onions, green peppers, thyme, ¼ teaspoon salt, and a few cracks of pepper. Cook for 10 minutes, stirring often. Add the garlic and cook another 5 minutes, or until the veggies are very soft.

Meanwhile, add the ground beef to a large bowl along with the eggs, Parmesan, 1 teaspoon salt, and a few cracks of pepper. Once the veggies are ready, add them to the bowl with the beef and use a large spoon to start mixing—the veggies will be too hot to handle. After mixing for 20 seconds, use your hands to thoroughly mix everything together, but make sure not too overmix or the meatloaf will be tough. Use a piece of wax paper or parchment paper and measure a nine-by-ten inch rectangle. Spread the meatloaf mixture onto the paper and shape it so it fits. Layer the cheese and prosciutto so they overlap on the meatloaf and then use the paper to roll the meatloaf up tightly. Pinch the ends of the meatloaf closed and flatten them, transfer meatloaf to a tin seam side down, and cover with as much keto ketchup as desired. If you don't have a meatloaf tin, place on a sheet tray, seam side down. Bake for roughly 75 minutes, or until the internal temperature is 155°F. Remove from oven and allow to cool for 10–20 minutes with some tin foil tented on top. Watch the YouTube video, it's not as hard as it sounds.

Make the veggies by cutting the eggplant and broccolini into large bite-size pieces and slice the shallots and garlic thinly. Pour 3 tablespoons of oil into a large non-stick pan and heat on medium-high for 2–3 minutes. Once hot, add the shallots, garlic, mustard seeds, and tilt the pan so they fry in the oil. Cook just until golden brown and then remove from pan but leave the oil behind. The shallots and garlic will burn easily, so make sure to pull them as soon as they are ready. Add the eggplant and broccolini to the pan, turn the heat up a notch, and cook for 5–7 minutes, or until the eggplant is golden brown and both veggies are cooked through. Add ¼ teaspoon of salt, a couple cracks of pepper, and turn off the heat. Mix well and add the lemon zest and juice. Check for seasoning as you may need more salt or lemon. Transfer the veggies to a clean bowl and top with the crispy shallots, garlic, and mustard seeds.

Slice the meatloaf, serve with the veggies, and enjoy!

STORAGE AND REHEATING: Everything will keep in the fridge for five days or can be frozen for two to three months. The best way to reheat everything is to thaw and place in a 350°F oven for 8–10 minutes. If using a microwave, make sure to cover the container with a wet paper towel and don't overheat the food or it will dry out.

MACROS

per serving of meatloaf (makes 5):
693 calories
3.1 grams of net carbs
5.5 grams of total carbs
50.2 grams of fat
47.6 grams of protein
0.6 grams of fiber

MACROS

per serving of veggies (makes 5):
132 calories
7.2 grams of net carbs
13 grams of total carbs
9.36 grams of fat
3.5 grams of protein
5.7 grams of fiber

★★★★★

"Just made this meatloaf recipe tonight! It was bomb dot com!!!! The flavors are on point! Def making this again." —**Lauren**

"The best meatloaf ever! Easy to make and full of flavor. The side dish is a perfect pairing." —**Lucia**

"I made this meatloaf today, and it turned out just perfect! Love the combination between beef and prosciutto and cheese and ahhh. It's just yummy!!" —**Benny**

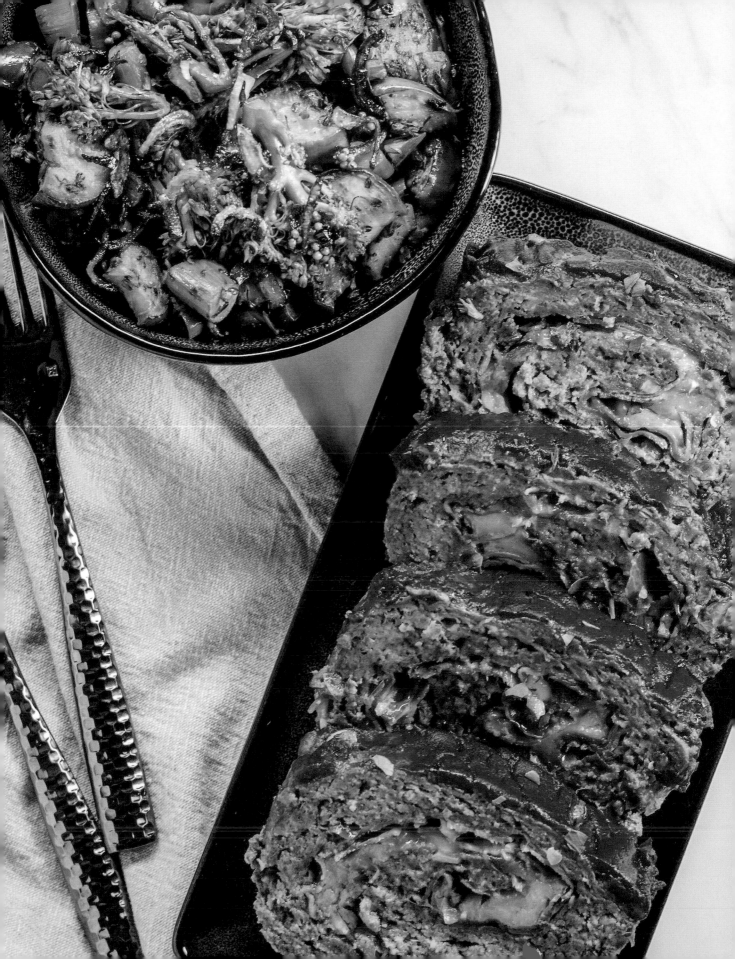

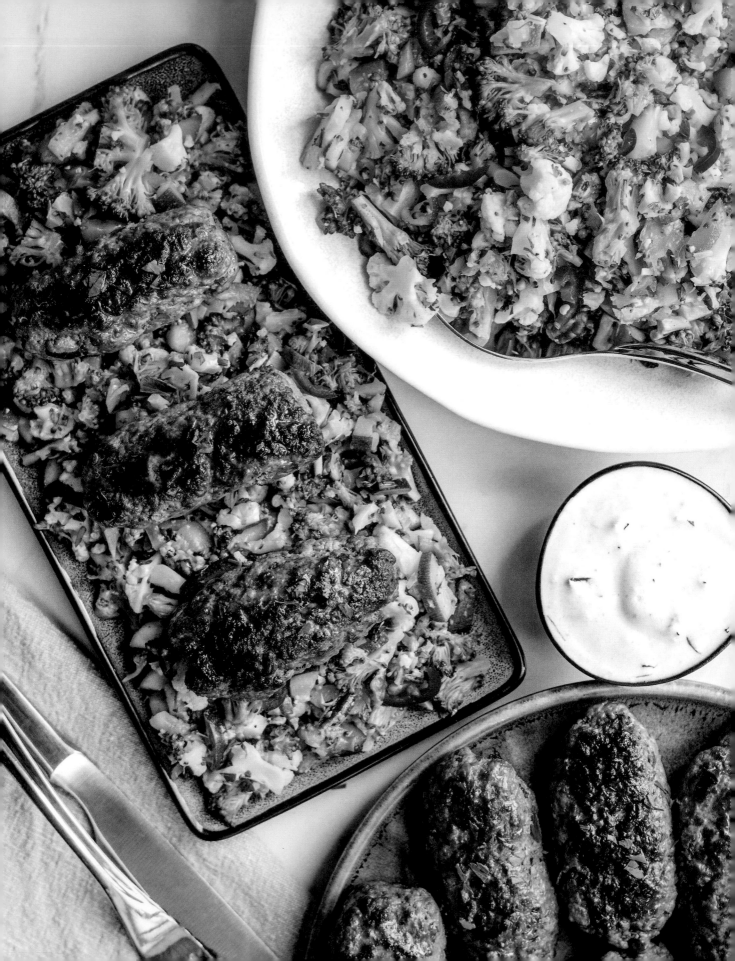

PREP TIME: **25 MINUTES** • COOKING TIME: **35 MINUTES** • MAKES: **5 MEALS**

BEEF KEFTA WITH VEGGIE PILAF
AND YOGURT SAUCE

This is my low-carb take on Middle Eastern comfort food. Instead of eating starchy rice, I use lots of keto-friendly veggies and the added crunch of pecans. The kefta are juicy and have the right blend of spices and herbs. Just don't forget to dip them in that creamy yogurt sauce.

FOR THE YOGURT SAUCE:
- ¾ cup full-fat Greek yogurt
- 1 teaspoon fresh parsley, chopped
- 1 teaspoon mint, chopped
- Zest of ½ lemon
- 1 tablespoon lemon juice
- 1 clove garlic
- 1 teaspoon extra virgin olive oil
- ¼ teaspoon kosher salt and black pepper

To watch the video tutorial for this recipe, search "FlavCity beef kefta" on YouTube.

FOR THE BEEF:
- 2 pounds ground beef, 80:20 beef to fat ratio
- 2 teaspoons fresh parsley, chopped
- 2 teaspoons mint, chopped
- 1½ teaspoons smoked paprika
- 1½ teaspoons cumin
- ¼ teaspoon cayenne pepper
- 2 cloves garlic, grated
- ½ teaspoon dried thyme
- Zest of ½ a lemon
- Kosher salt and fresh pepper
- Avocado oil

FOR THE PILAF:
- 2 medium-sized zucchinis, about 12 ounces
- 1 head of cauliflower
- 1 pound of broccoli with stalks or 12 ounces of florets
- ½ onion, chopped
- 2 cloves garlic, minced
- 1 teaspoon mustard seeds
- ¼ teaspoon red pepper flakes
- 1 teaspoon fresh parsley, chopped
- 1 teaspoon mint, chopped
- Zest and juice of ½ lemon
- 2 tablespoons chopped pecans, roasted if desired
- Kosher salt and fresh pepper
- Avocado oil

Make the pilaf by chopping the zucchini, cauliflower, and broccoli into small pieces that are roughly the same size, making sure not to use too much of the stalks. Preheat a large non-stick pan over medium heat for 2 minutes. Add 1 tablespoon of oil to the pan and then the onions, garlic, mustard seeds, red pepper flakes, ¼ teaspoon salt, and a couple cracks of pepper. Mix well and cook for 6 minutes, stirring often. Add the chopped zucchini, cauliflower, and broccoli to the pan along with ½ teaspoon of salt and a few cracks of pepper. Mix well and place a lid on the pan. You can also use a sheet tray to cover the pan if you don't have a lid. Cook for 10–12 minutes, stirring a few times. The veggies are ready when they have softened up, but still have a bite to them. Turn the heat off the pan and add the parsley, mint, lemon zest and juice, and pecans, and mix well. Check for seasoning as you may need more lemon juice or salt. Set aside.

For the beef kefta, add the ground beef to a large bowl along with the remaining ingredients (except the oil), 1 teaspoon of salt, and a few cracks of pepper. Use your hands to mix everything well, making sure not to overmix. Form the kefta by taking a little of the meat and shaping it like log or football. You will have enough beef to make 14 15 kefta. Preheat a large pan, preferably cast-iron, just above medium heat for 2 minutes. Add 1 tablespoon of oil to the pan, wait 30 seconds so the oil can heat up, and then add half the kefta to the pan. Cook for 3–4 minutes or until well browned and flip and cook another 3–4 minutes. Once both sides are browned, you may need to cook the kefta on the sides for 30 seconds to cook them all the way through. If you are not sure the kefta are done, cut one in half and check as it's important not to overcook them. Otherwise, they will dry out. Remove kefta from pan, add more oil, and cook the second batch.

While the kefta are cooking, **make the yogurt sauce** by combining everything in a bowl and whisking well. Check for seasoning and adjust if needed.

Serve the kefta with some yogurt sauce and pilaf and enjoy!

STORAGE AND REHEATING: Everything will keep in the fridge for five days. You can freeze the kefta for two to three months, but I would not recommend freezing the veggies as they will get very soft and watery. The best way to reheat the kefta and veggies is in a 350°F oven for 7–10 minutes. If using a microwave, cover the container with a wet paper towel and make sure not to overheat, as the beef will dry out.

MACROS

**per serving of kefta
(each serving is 3 kefta):**
401 calories
0.40 grams of net and total carbs
28.8 grams of fat
30.7 grams of protein
0 fiber

MACROS

for all the yogurt sauce:
168 calories
7.5 net and total grams of carbs
12.4 grams of fat
16 grams of protein
0 fiber

MACROS

**per serving of pilaf
(makes 5):**
91 calories
8 grams of net carbs
14.5 grams of total carbs
4 grams of fat
4.4 grams of protein
6.3 grams of fiber

★★★★★

"Made this meal yesterday with ground chuck, and ohhhh did it turn out delicious!! Basically, have been learning how to cook this summer solely by using your recipes and videos." **—Christopher L.**

PREP TIME: **20 MINUTES** • COOK TIME: **1 HOUR 40 MINUTES** • MAKES: **6 STUFFED PEPPERS**

BEEFY STUFFED PEPPERS
WITH TOMATO SAUCE

Why do most stuffed pepper recipes call for cooking the filling before baking in the oven? Do people like overcooked beef and raw peppers? This recipe ensures the beef and pork filling is cooked perfectly while the peppers have long enough to cook down and soften.

To watch the video tutorial for this recipe, search "FlavCity stuffed peppers" on YouTube.

INGREDIENTS:

- ½ onion, diced
- 1 medium-sized zucchini, diced
- ½ teaspoon dried thyme
- 6 bell peppers
- ¼ cup walnuts, chopped
- 2 cloves garlic, minced
- 1 tablespoon tomato paste
- ½ teaspoon smoked paprika
- ½ teaspoon cumin
- ¼ teaspoon cayenne pepper
- ⅓ cup chicken stock/broth
- ¾ pound ground beef
- ¾ pound ground pork
- 1 egg
- 1 twenty-eight-ounce can tomato puree, unsalted
- 1 cup shredded cheddar cheese
- ½ cup grated Parmesan cheese
- Kosher salt and fresh pepper
- Avocado oil

Preheat oven to 350°F. **For the filling,** preheat a large non-stick pan just above medium heat along with 1 tablespoon of oil. Add the onions, zucchini, thyme, ½ teaspoon salt, and a few cracks of pepper and mix well. Cook for 10 minutes, stirring often. Meanwhile, cut the tops of the bell peppers off and use your hands to carefully rip out the seeds and membranes.

Add the walnuts, garlic, tomato paste, smoked paprika, cumin, and cayenne to the onion mixture and cook for 3 minutes, stirring often. Add the chicken stock to the pan and cook for 1 minute, or until most of the liquid is absorbed and the mixture looks wet. Set aside.

Place the ground beef and pork in a large bowl, season with 1 teaspoon of salt, a few cracks of pepper, and add the egg. Add the veggie mixture to the beef and use your hands or a large spoon if the veggies are still hot in order to mix everything until combined. It's ok that the veggies are hot because you will be cooking the peppers immediately, but, if that is not the case, make sure the veggies cool before adding to the meat.

Add the tomato puree to a baking dish along with ½ teaspoon of salt and few cracks of pepper, mix well, and then add the bell peppers. Use a spoon to stuff the peppers to the top, making sure to pack the onion and meat mixture down. Cover the baking dish with tin foil, place on a sheet tray and bake for 30 minutes. Remove tin foil and bake another 30 minutes.

For the cheesy topping, combine the cheddar cheese and Parmesan in a bowl and mix well. After the peppers have been cooking for one hour, top them with the cheese and and bake uncovered for another 25–30 minutes. If you have a thermometer, remove the peppers from the oven when internal temperature is 155°F.

Allow the peppers to rest for 10–20 minutes before serving, plate them up with some reserved tomato sauce, enjoy!

STORAGE AND REHEATING: The peppers will keep in the fridge for five days and get even better the second and third day. You can freeze the stuffed peppers for three months. Thaw and reheat in a 350°F oven for 10 minutes.

MACROS

per pepper (makes 6):
494 calories
6.5 grams of net carbs
9.6 grams of total carbs
37.1 grams of fat
30.2 grams of protein
2.8 grams of fiber

MACROS

for every ¼ cup of tomato sauce:
18 calories
4.4 grams of net carbs
5.6 grams of total carbs
Less than 1 gram of fat
1.1 grams of fiber
0.93 grams of protein

★★★★★

"This is a flavor-packed, delicious, and visually beautiful dish. I had visitors that are on the keto diet, and I wanted to make a couple of dishes that they would feel comfortable eating. They really enjoyed these. I also like that these are highly customizable, though they are so good if you follow the recipe. Will definitely make these again. Keep dishes like this coming guys." **—Arlene B.**

"My husband and I watched your keto stuffed peppers video, and our mouths were watering watching it. So we made your recipe two nights ago, and they are AMAZINGLY delish! They are definitely packed with flavor and shockingly filling. We ate leftovers last night, and they were even better than the first night. There is only one pepper left, and I am going to savor every last bite today. That is the first recipe of yours that we have tried, as we have just recently discovered FlavCity. If all of your keto recipes are this tasty, then you can expect two new devoted followers here. Thanks!" **—Erik and Monica**

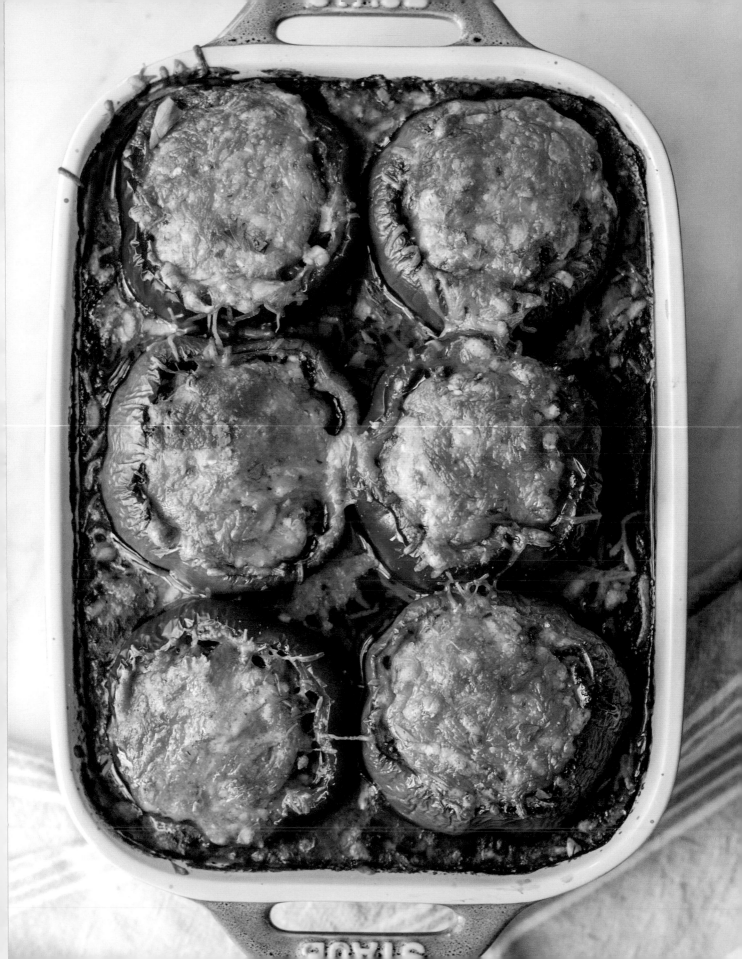

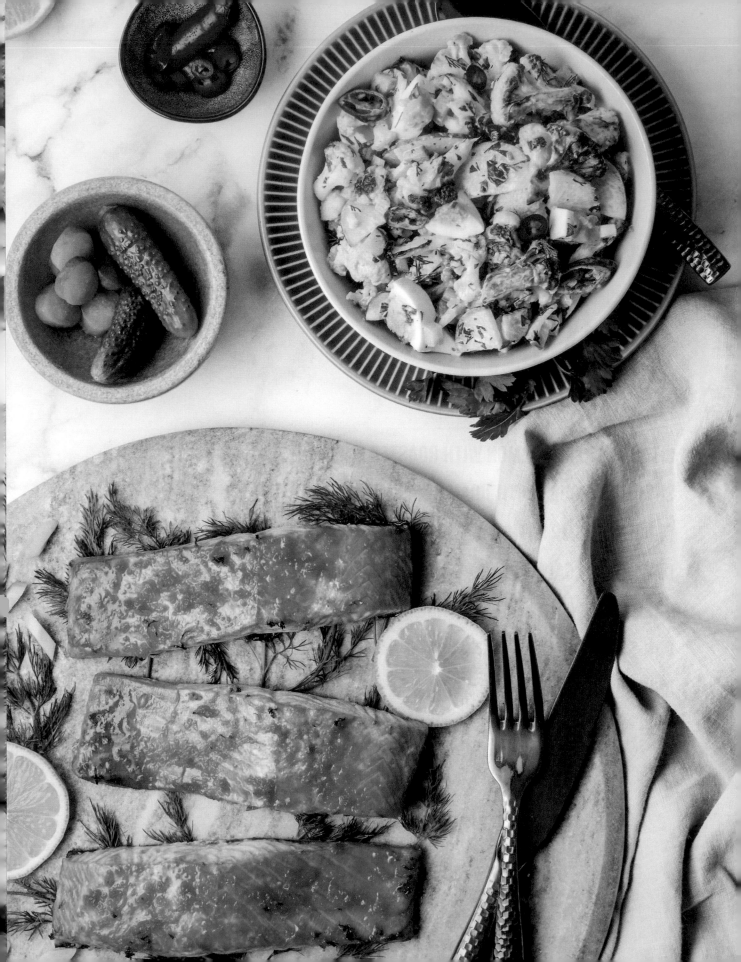

PREP TIME: **20 MINUTES** • COOKING TIME: **60 MINUTES** • MAKES: **5 MEALS**

CITRUS-GLAZED SALMON
WITH ROASTED CAULIFLOWER SALAD

One of the most popular requests on my YouTube channel is for lunch recipes that can be eaten cold at work and school. You will definitely make your buddies envious of your lunch when you break out this juicy brown sugar and citrus glazed salmon with loaded cauliflower salad.

 Tip | Cooked salmon will only keep in the fridge for three days. Plan on freezing two of the cooked or raw pieces for a later date.

 | To watch the video tutorial for this recipe, search "FlavCity salmon and cauliflower" on YouTube.

FOR THE SALMON:

- 5 salmon filets, 5–6 ounces each
- 5 tablespoons brown sugar substitute, like Sukrin Gold
- 2 lemons
- 1 large orange
- Kosher salt

FOR THE CAULIFLOWER SALAD:

- 1 large head of cauliflower
- 1 teaspoon dried thyme
- 2 eggs
- 3 dill pickles, chopped
- 2 stalks celery, chopped
- 5 radishes, thinly sliced
- 2 tablespoons parsley, finely chopped
- 2 tablespoons fresh dill, finely chopped
- 1 long red finger chili, finely sliced
- Avocado or olive oil
- Kosher salt and fresh pepper

FOR THE DRESSING:

- ½ cup full-fat, sugar-free mayonnaise
- ½ teaspoon sesame oil
- 1 teaspoon tamari soy sauce
- Zest and juice of ½ lemon
- Kosher salt and fresh pepper

Prep the salmon by seasoning the top of each salmon filet with the 1 tablespoon of brown sugar substitute, some lemon and orange zest, and a nice pinch of salt. Place in the fridge for 30–60 minutes.

Meanwhile, start on the salad. Preheat oven to 450°F and chop the cauliflower into large bite-size florets. Place the cauliflower on a sheet tray and season with 1 tablespoon of oil, dried thyme, just under 1 teaspoon salt, and a few cracks of pepper. Cook in the oven for 30 minutes or until the cauliflower is well browned.

While the cauliflower cooks, bring a medium-sized pot of water to a boil and cook the eggs. To get beautiful yellow egg yolks, turn the heat down to a simmer as soon as the eggs go in the water and cook for exactly 12 minutes. Remove eggs, run under cold water, peel, and chop. In a large bowl, add the chopped eggs, pickles, chili, celery, radishes, and herbs. Once the cauliflower is roasted, carefully add it to the bowl.

Make the dressing by combining everything in a small bowl along with a ¼ teaspoon of salt and a few cracks of pepper and whisking well. Check for seasoning. You may need more lemon juice as you want the flavor to be nice and tart. Add almost all the dressing to the salad and mix well, adding more dressing if needed. Taste for seasoning and set aside.

To cook the salmon, preheat the broiler to high and make sure the oven rack is eight to ten inches away from the broiling element. Remove the salmon from the fridge and place them on a sheet tray lined with tin foil, making sure no excess glaze is on the foil. Otherwise, it will burn and smoke. Broil the salmon for 6–8 minutes until the top is well browned and the fish feels firm when pinched on the sides. Since it's hard to know when salmon is ready and the last thing you want to do is overcook it, just cut one piece in half and see if it is done to your liking. Remove from oven.

Plate the salmon with the salad and enjoy!

STORAGE AND REHEATING: The cauliflower salad will keep in the fridge for five days but can't be frozen. The salmon will keep in the fridge for three days or can be frozen for two months. It's best to thaw the salmon the night before and reheat in a 350°F oven for 7–10 minutes. If reheating in a microwave, cover the dish with a wet paper towel and make sure not dry out the salmon.

Keto Meal Prep

MACROS

per serving of salmon (makes 5):

295 calories

0 net carbs and total (erythritol does not affect blood sugar)

19 grams of fat

29 grams of protein

0 fiber

MACROS

per serving of salad (makes 5):

236 calories

3.2 grams of net carbs

5.4 grams of total carbs

21 grams of fat

4.3 grams of protein

3.8 grams of fiber

★★★★★

"Thanks for this recipe, Bobby! My husband loves it. It's perfect with this high heat we're having in California. I love how it only took one hour out of my Sunday to prep a week's worth of lunch." —**Maria L.**

"Bobby! I made this last night! So perfect for my work week lunch. BUUTT...I took one bite of the roasted cauliflower, and I ended up eating half of the tray!!! It was sooooo good! I'm addicted." —**Lifestyle My Style**

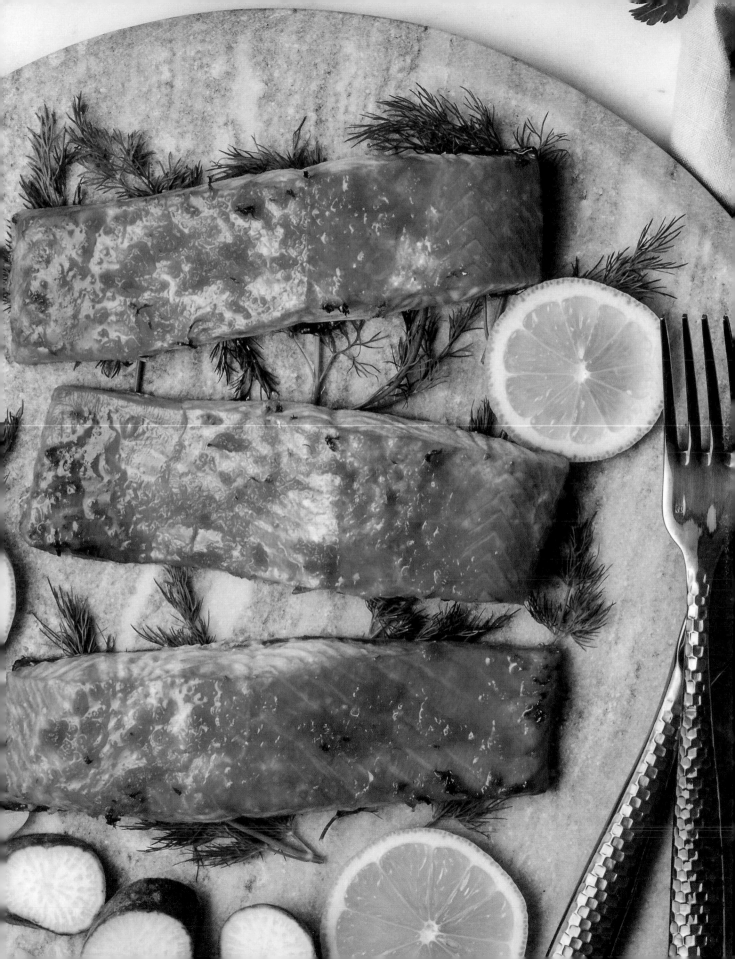

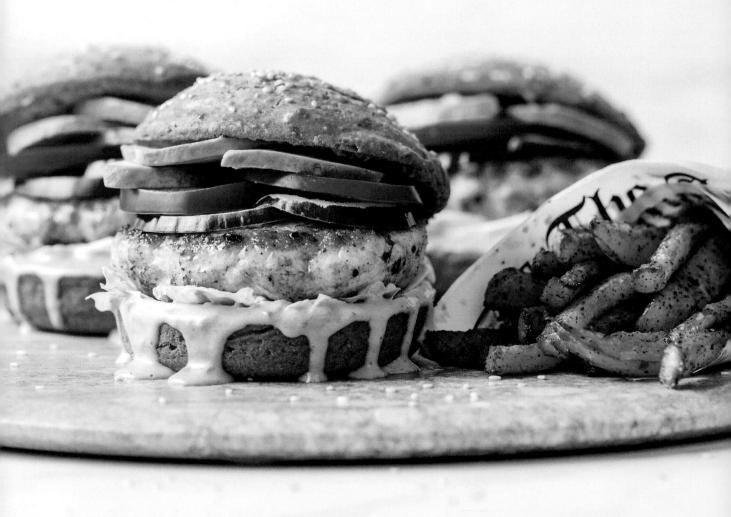

PREP TIME: **30 MINUTES** • COOKING TIME: **45 MINUTES** • MAKES: **5 MEALS**   PALEO

SHRIMP BURGERS
WITH JICAMA FRIES AND SECRET SAUCE

Shrimp burgers, who does that!? Me, that's who! Just look at that photo: the burgers are juicy, loaded with flavor, and even better tasting than they look! A burger needs some fries, and these smoky spiced jicama fries do the trick.

FOR THE BUNS:
- See recipe for Keto Fat Bread on page 161

Tip | While jicama is much lower in carbs than potatoes, they should be eaten in moderation on the keto diet. This recipe makes enough for five small servings. You can buy pre-chopped jicama at Trader Joe's—this will save you some prep time.

Tip | You can use iceberg lettuce as the bun. It's crispy and will save you some time instead of making the buns.

 | To watch the video tutorial for this recipe, search "FlavCity shrimp burger" on YouTube.

FOR THE SECRET SAUCE:
- ⅓ cup full-fat, sugar-free mayonnaise
- 3 tablespoons keto ketchup, no sugar added
- 1 tablespoon dill relish, no sugar added
- ¾ teaspoon tabasco sauce
- 1 tablespoon fresh lemon juice
- ¼ teaspoon kosher salt and couple cracks of fresh pepper

FOR THE JICAMA FRIES:
- 2 pounds jicama
- ½ teaspoon cumin
- ½ teaspoon smoked paprika
- ¼ teaspoon cayenne pepper
- Avocado or olive oil
- Kosher salt

FOR THE SHRIMP BURGERS:
- 2 pounds shrimp, shells off and cleaned
- 2 tablespoons full-fat, sugar-free mayonnaise
- Zest of ½ lemon
- 1½ teaspoons capers, drained
- 1 heaping teaspoon stone-ground or Dijon mustard
- 1 teaspoon onion powder
- 1 teaspoon garlic powder
- ¼ cup thinly sliced green onions
- 1 teaspoon kosher salt and few cracks of fresh pepper
- Avocado or olive oil
- Toppings of your choice

For the burgers, add ⅛ of the shrimp to a food processor and puree until smooth. Add the rest of the shrimp and the remaining burger ingredients up until and including the salt and pepper and puree until almost smooth—you want a little texture. The way I like to form burger patties is to divide the mixture into five portions, put a piece of plastic wrap over a large peanut butter jar lid (3.5 inches wide), add a portion of the shrimp mixture to the lid, pack it down, and lift the plastic wrap out. Finish forming the burger using your hands and move to a plate or platter. Repeat with remaining shrimp mixture. Place the burgers in the fridge for 30 minutes. This will help the mixture set up, so the burgers don't fall apart.

For the keto buns, follow the instruction for Keto Fat Bread on page 161 to make the batter. You will need to buy a hamburger bun tin that is 1.5 inches deep. I use one from Amazon called "USA pan bakeware mini round cake pans." When the buns come out from the oven, they may have a pointed dome. Rest a ramekin on top, and it will push the buns down and make them look good.

Meanwhile, **start the fries** by preheating the oven to 425°F and bringing a medium-sized pot of water to a boil. Peel the jicama with a veggie peeler then slice them into long fries about ¼ inch thick. Add 1 teaspoon of salt to the boiling water along with the fries. Boil for 15 minutes. Drain fries and pat them completely dry with a large towel. Place fries on a sheet tray and season with 1–2 tablespoons of oil, ¾ teaspoon salt, smoked paprika, cumin, cayenne pepper, and mix very well using your hands. Arrange the fries in one layer and bake in the oven for 35 minutes. Turn the broiler to high and broil for another 5–10 minutes until the fries have some color on all sides.

Make the secret sauce by combining everything in a small bowl and whisking well. Check for seasoning and set aside.

Make the burgers by preheating a large non-stick pan over medium-high heat for 2 minutes. Add 1 tablespoon of oil, wait 30 seconds so the oil can heat up, and then add 3–4 burgers. You can't overcrowd the pan, so cook the burgers in two batches. Cook for 4–5 minutes, or until a nice golden-brown crust has formed, flip, and cook no longer than 4 minutes more. You know the burgers are ready when you press in the middle and they feel firm with a little give. Repeat process with the second batch.

Griddle the buns with some butter in a non-stick pan until golden and serve the burger with toppings of your choice and fries. Enjoy!

STORAGE AND REHEATING: Shrimp burgers will keep in the fridge for three or four days or can be frozen for two to three months. Jicama fries will keep in the fridge for five days but can't be frozen. The best way to reheat everything is in a 350°F oven for 7–10 minutes or in a microwave. Just make sure to cover the container with a wet paper towel and don't overheat the shrimp or it will get dry.

MACROS	per burger patty (makes 5)	MACROS	for all the special sauce:	MACROS	per bun (makes 5):	MACROS	per serving of fries (makes 5):
	256 calories		560 calories		566 calories		118 calories
	1.64 grams of net and total carbs		6 grams of net and total carbs		5 grams of net carbs		7 grams of net carbs
					13.2 grams of total carbs		16 grams of total carbs
	9.9 grams of fat		58 grams of fat		52.2 grams of fat		5.8 grams of fat
	31 grams of protein		1 gram of protein		10.8 grams of protein		1.3 grams of protein
	0 fiber		0 fiber		8 grams of fiber		9 grams of fiber

★★★★★

"The shrimp burgers are delicious! Definitely will make again! Bomb.com lol" —**Maddie**

"Bobby, I made this tonight and was stunned—I mean absolutely astounded—by how delicious and easy this was to make. I just want anyone out here listening that FlavCity recipes deliver incredible taste, simplicity, and variety. Thank you, Bobby, for continuing to bless the low-carb, keto community." —**Leyonna**

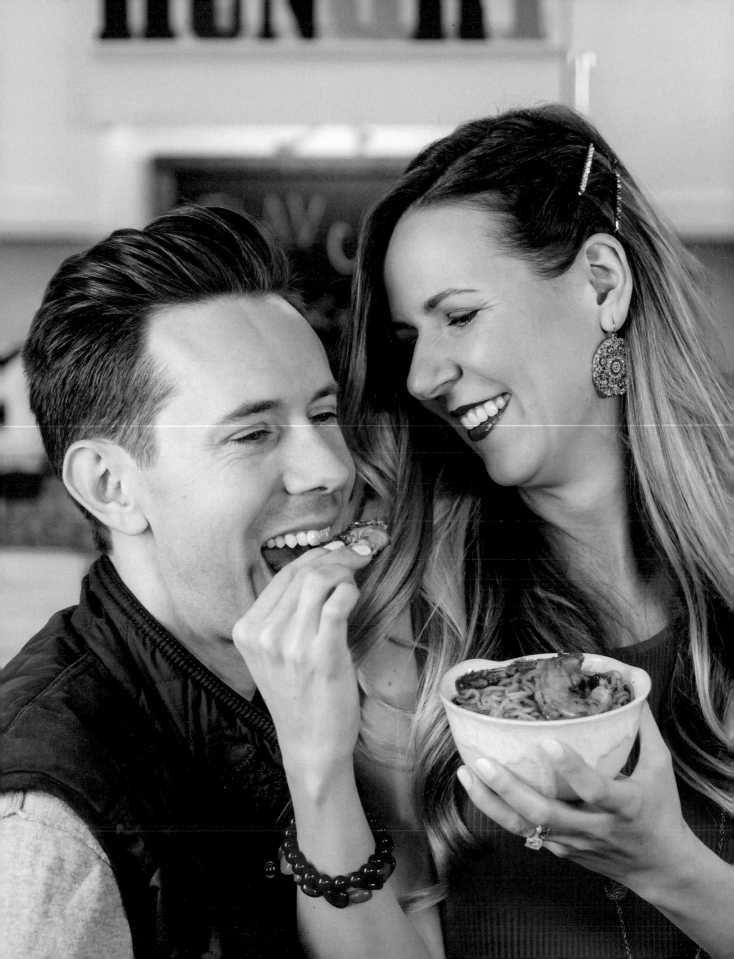

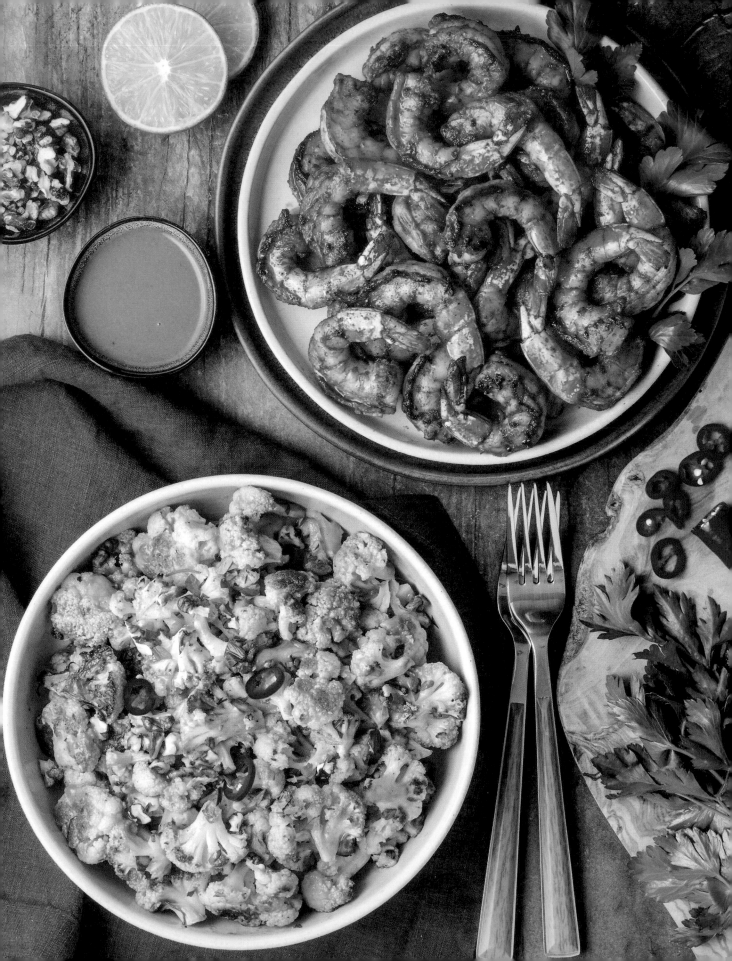

PREP TIME: **20 MINUTES** • COOKING TIME: **40 MINUTES** • MAKES: **5 MEALS**

PALEO / WHOLE30

CRUSTY SHRIMP
WITH ROASTED CAULIFLOWER CURRY

This creamy coconut curry sauce is one of my favorite things to make. You could pour it over cardboard and it would taste good, but I much prefer oven-roasted cauliflower served with juicy spice-crusted shrimp.

 Tip | Cooked shrimp will only keep in the fridge for three days. Either freeze some of the cooked shrimp or buy more later in the week.

FOR THE CAULIFLOWER:

- 1½ large heads of cauliflower
- 2 teaspoons fresh thyme, chopped
- 3 tablespoons walnuts, roasted and chopped
- Fresh cilantro or parsley, chopped
- Kosher salt and fresh pepper
- Avocado oil

FOR THE CURRY SAUCE:

- ½ onion, chopped
- 2 cloves garlic, minced
- 1½ teaspoons freshly grated ginger
- 1 small red chili, finely sliced or a pinch of pepper flakes
- 2 teaspoons yellow curry powder
- 1 teaspoon turmeric powder
- ¾ cup full-fat coconut milk
- ⅓ cup chicken or veggie stock
- 1 teaspoon lime juice
- 2 tablespoons coconut cream
- Kosher salt and fresh pepper
- Avocado or olive oil

FOR THE SHRIMP:

- 2 pounds shrimp, cleaned with tails on
- 1 teaspoon smoked paprika
- 1 teaspoon turmeric
- 1 teaspoon cumin
- Kosher salt
- Avocado oil

To roast the cauliflower, preheat oven to 450°F and chop the cauliflower into large bite-size florets. Place the cauliflower on a sheet tray and drizzle 2 tablespoons of avocado oil, 1 teaspoon salt, a few cracks of pepper, and the thyme (use ½ teaspoon if using dried thyme) onto the cauliflower. Toss to combine and roast in the oven for 30 minutes, until well browned on all sides.

Make the curry sauce by preheating a medium-sized pan over medium heat for 2 minutes. Add 2 teaspoons of oil to the pan along with the onions, ¼ teaspoon salt, a couple cracks pepper, and mix well. Cook for 8 minutes, then add the ginger, chili, and garlic. Cook for 3 minutes, then add the curry powder and turmeric; mix well, and cook for 1 more minute, stirring often. Add the coconut milk, chicken stock, ¼ teaspoon of salt, bring to a boil and then reduce to a simmer. Let simmer for 12 minutes or until reduced by half and has a saucy consistency. Turn off the heat, add the lime juice and check for seasoning as you may need more lime juice. Stir in the coconut cream and then strain the sauce into a bowl so it's silky and smooth. You can also blend the sauce instead of straining, if desired.

Once the cauliflower is ready, place it in a medium-sized bowl and pour on just enough curry sauce to thoroughly coat. Add the walnuts and cilantro, toss well, and check for seasoning. Set aside.

For the shrimp, use paper towels to pat the shrimp as dry as possible. Make the spice rub by combing the smoked paprika, turmeric, and cumin in a small bowl and mix well. Season the shrimp with 1 teaspoon of salt and enough spice rub to coat, along with 1 teaspoon of oil and mix well with your hands. Preheat a large non-stick or cast-iron pan just under high heat for 2 minutes and then add 2 teaspoons of oil and wait 30 seconds. Add half the shrimp to the pan and cook for 2 minutes, flip, cook another 2 minutes, and then remove from the pan. Repeat with second batch.

Serve the shrimp with the cauliflower and any leftover curry sauce. Enjoy!

STORAGE AND REHEATING: Cooked shrimp will only last in the fridge for three days, so either freeze some or cook another batch later in the week. To reheat, thaw the shrimp first and then warm with the cauliflower in a 350°F oven for 6–8 minutes. You can also toss in a hot pan for 1 minute. If using the microwave, cover the open container with a wet paper towel and make sure not to overheat or the shrimp will dry out.

MACROS

per serving of cauliflower (makes 5):
201 calories
5.4 grams of net carbs
8.3 grams of total carbs
16.3 grams of fat
2.8 grams of protein
5.3 grams of fiber

MACROS

per serving of shrimp (makes 5):
216 calories
1.6 grams of net and total carbs
5.9 grams of fat
37 grams of protein
0 fiber

PREP TIME: **25 MINUTES** • COOKING TIME: **40 MINUTES** • MAKES: **5 MEALS**

CRISPY SKIN SALMON
WITH BLISTERED SNOW PEAS AND RICE PILAF

If you are looking for new ways to cook salmon, here you go. This technique will give you insanely crispy skin, but the fish will be juicy and moist. The side dishes are actually my favorite part of the recipe: so much flavor and so many veggies!

 Tip | Cooked salmon will only keep in the fridge for three days, so plan on freezing two of the filets.

 | To watch a similar video tutorial for this recipe, search "FlavCity salmon meal prep" on YouTube.

FOR THE SALMON:
- 5 salmon filets, 6 ounces each
- Avocado oil
- Kosher salt and fresh pepper

FOR THE CAULIFLOWER RICE PILAF:
- See recipe on page 179

FOR THE SNOW PEAS:
- 12 ounces snow peas
- ½ cup red onion, finely sliced
- 2 cloves garlic, minced
- ½ red chili, finely sliced or ¼ teaspoon red pepper flakes
- 1½ tablespoon tamari soy sauce
- ½ teaspoon toasted sesame oil
- 1 teaspoon sesame seeds
- Avocado oil
- Kosher salt and fresh pepper

Prep the salmon by placing the salmon filets skin side up on a plate and storing in the fridge 30–60 minutes before cooking.

Make the cauliflower rice pilaf by using the recipe on page 179.

For the blistered snow peas, preheat a large-sized non-stick pan just below high heat for 2 minutes. Add 2 teaspoons of oil along with the snow peas. Cook for 3–4 minutes, mixing often until blistered and charred in spots on the exterior, but still crunchy. Add the onions, garlic, chili, ¼ teaspoon salt, couple cracks of pepper, and cook for 1 minute. Add the tamari, sesame oil, and sesame seeds, and cook for 1 minute more. Transfer to a bowl and check for seasoning, as you may need a bit more sesame oil or tamari.

For the salmon, preheat a non-stick pan over medium-high heat for 2 minutes along with 2 teaspoons of oil. You will have to work in batches to cook the salmon as you don't want to overcrowd the pan. Season the skin side of the salmon filets with a generous pinch of salt and a couple cracks of pepper. Place the salmon filets in the pan, skin side down, and gently press down on them for 5 seconds to make sure they are making maximum contact with the pan. Season the top side of the salmon with another pinch of salt and some pepper. Cook the salmon skin side down for 4–5 minutes or until the skin is deep golden brown and the sides of the fish are white. Use a spatula and flip the filets and immediately lower the heat just below medium and cook for another 3 minutes. After 3 minutes, turn the salmon on the fleshy side and cook for 30 seconds, repeat on the other side. This will ensure the salmon cooks through evenly. Remove from the pan and repeat with remaining salmon.

Serve the salmon filet with some cauliflower rice and snow peas and enjoy!

STORAGE AND REHEATING: Cauliflower rice and snow peas will keep in the fridge for five days and the salmon will only last three days. Salmon can be frozen for two to three months, but I don't recommend freezing the veggies as they will get very mushy when they thaw. Reheat in a 350°F oven for 10 minutes or cover the food with a wet paper towel and gently reheat in microwave, making sure to not overheat the food or it will get dry.

Keto Meal Prep

MACROS

per salmon filet:

295 calories
0 carbs
19 grams of fat
29 grams of protein
0 fiber

MACROS

per serving of pilaf (makes 5):

76 calories
7.6 grams of net carbs
12.4 grams of total carbs
2.6 grams of fat
4.9 grams of protein
4.2 grams of fiber

MACROS

per serving of snow peas (makes 5):

40 calories
5.2 grams of net carbs
7.1 grams of total carbs
2.5 grams of fat
2 grams of protein
1.8 grams of fiber

★★★★★

"Made the main dish. I just moved out and I thought I hated salmon, but it turns out I just don't like the way my mom made it. Thank you so much! This was delish!!" —**Mickey L.**

"Omg, I made the cauliflower rice dish and the salmon. So awesome!!!!" —**TheJanicetunes**

"Omg! I made the rice and salmon sooooooo amazingly delish!!!" —**Xochitl M.**

"Just made it today and it was DELICIOUS!!!" —**Ana M.**

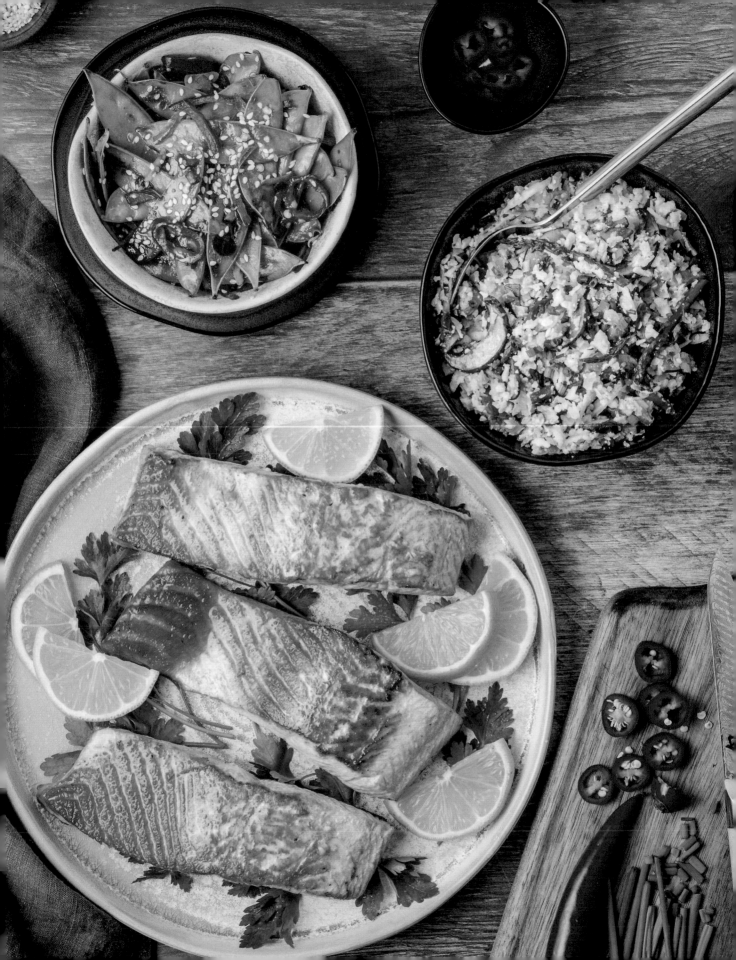

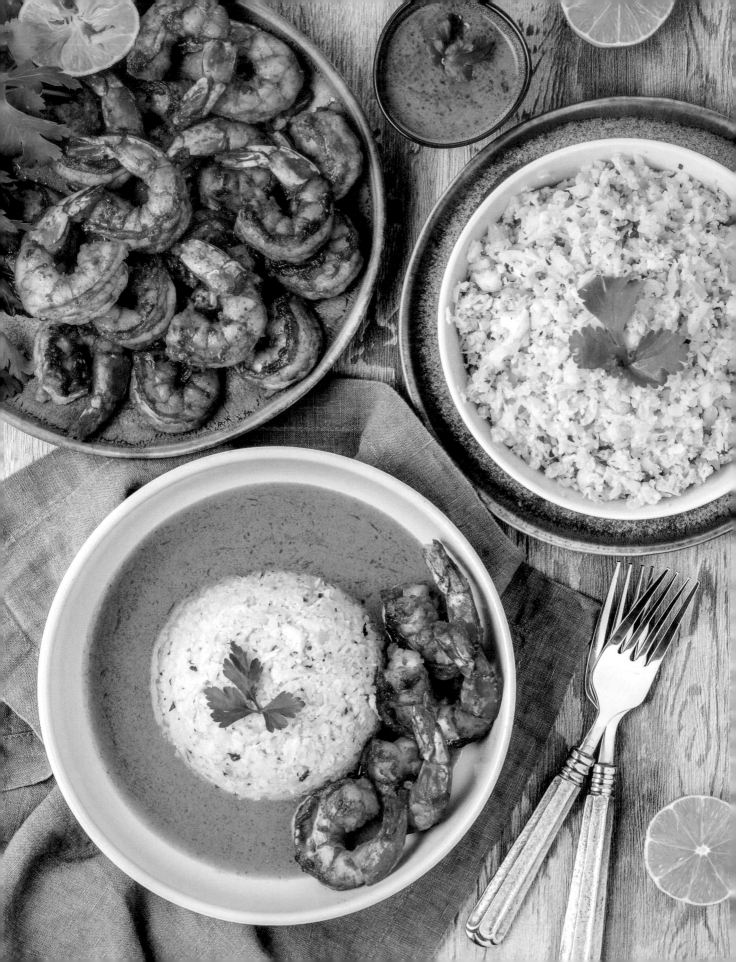

PREP TIME: **10 MINUTES** • COOKING TIME: **25 MINUTES** • MAKES: **5 MEALS**

PALEO / WHOLE30

GREEN CURRY SHRIMP
WITH CAULIFLOWER RICE

It only takes six fresh ingredients to make this stunner of a recipe. The secret is a jar of green curry paste from the store. It's loaded with ginger, lemongrass, and chilies which will help add big flavors with minimal effort. Every curry needs a proper rice to soak up the goodness. This cauliflower rice is about as easy as they get.

 To watch the video tutorial for this recipe, search "FlavCity green curry shrimp" on YouTube.

INGREDIENTS:
- 2 pounds large shrimp, peeled and deveined
- 1 teaspoon turmeric powder
- 1 teaspoon smoked paprika
- ½ teaspoon cayenne pepper
- ½ cup red onions, finely chopped
- 3 cloves garlic, minced
- 2 tablespoons green curry paste
- 1 can (13.5 ounces) full-fat coconut milk
- ¼ cup chicken stock or water
- Zest and juice of 1 lime
- 5 cups cauliflower rice, about 1 large head of cauliflower
- ¼ cup fresh cilantro, chopped
- Avocado oil
- Kosher salt and fresh pepper

Prep the shrimp by patting them dry and adding them to a large bowl with 1 teaspoon of oil. Make the spice rub by combining the paprika, turmeric, and cayenne pepper in a small bowl. Add the spice rub to the shrimp, mix well, and keep in the fridge until ready to cook.

Start the curry sauce by preheating a non-stick pan just above medium heat along with 1 tablespoon of oil for 2 minutes. Add the onion, ¼ teaspoon salt, and a couple cracks of pepper, and mix well. Cook for 6 minutes and then add the garlic. Cook another 4 minutes and then add the curry paste and cook for 1 minute. Add the coconut milk and chicken stock to the pan along with the zest and juice of half a lime and ¼ teaspoon salt. Bring the milk to a simmer and allow to reduce by almost half. Check for seasoning; you may need more lime juice and/or salt. Set aside. If you want to make the curry sauce very green, boil a small handful of cilantro for 1 minute, then blend it with a splash of reserved cooking water in the blender, and add that to the curry sauce. This is totally optional and only for obsessive people like me! Pass the sauce through a strainer into a measuring cup and set aside.

Make the cauliflower rice by preheating a large non-stick pan just above medium heat with 2 teaspoons of oil for 2 minutes. Add the cauliflower rice along with ½ teaspoon salt, a few cracks of pepper, and mix well. Cook for 5–7 minutes or until the raw flavor is gone from the veggies, but they still have a little bite. Add the zest and juice of half a lime and the cilantro, then check for seasoning. You may need more lime juice.

Cook the shrimp by preheating the same non-stick pan, or better yet use a large, cast-iron skillet over medium-high heat for 3 minutes. Add 1 tablespoon of oil to the pan and then half the shrimp. Cook for 2 minutes on each side and remove from pan. Add another shot of oil and cook the second batch of shrimp.

Serve the shrimp with cauliflower rice and pour over some curry sauce. Enjoy!

STORAGE AND REHEATING: Shrimp will keep in the fridge for three days or can be frozen for two to three months. Cauliflower rice and curry sauce will keep in the fridge for five days or can be frozen for two to three months. Thaw and reheat the shrimp in a 350°F oven for 7–10 minutes or gently reheat in the microwave, covered with a wet paper towel.

MACROS

per serving of shrimp and sauce (makes 5):
379 calories
5.1 grams of net carbs
6.2 grams of total carbs
21.1 grams of fat
38.1 grams of protein
0.6 fiber

MACROS

per serving of cauliflower rice (makes 5):
47 calories
3.3 grams of net carbs
5.5 grams of total carbs
2.3 grams of fat
2.1 grams of protein
2.2 grams of fiber

PREP TIME: **15 MINUTES** • COOKING TIME: **25 MINUTES** • MAKES: **3 MEALS**

PALEO / WHOLE30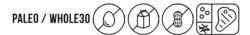

PAN-SEARED SALMON
WITH WILTED KALE AND MUSHROOMS

We make salmon at least once a week at home, and this recipe shows you a technique for making some of the crispiest skin you will ever eat! Best of all, this meal prep will take you less than 30 minutes to make and the flavors are top notch.

 Tip | To achieve that crispy skin on the salmon, let the salmon sit in the fridge skin side up for at 30–60 minutes before cooking. The goal is to dry out the skin, which helps make it crispy.

 | To watch the video tutorial for this recipe, search "FlavCity keto salmon" on YouTube.

FOR THE SALMON:
- 3 salmon filets, 5–6 ounces each
- Kosher salt
- Avocado oil

FOR THE KALE:
- 12 ounces cremini/baby bella mushrooms
- 1 bunch black (lacinato) kale
- ½ red onion, diced
- ¼ teaspoon red pepper flakes
- 2 cloves garlic, minced
- ¼ cup chicken stock or water
- Zest of ½ lemon
- 1 teaspoon lemon juice
- Kosher salt and fresh pepper
- Olive or avocado oil

FOR THE TOMATO SALAD:
- 1½ cups cherry tomatoes, quartered
- ½ cup radishes, thinly sliced
- 1 teaspoon fresh parsley or basil, chopped
- 1 tablespoon extra virgin olive oil
- ¼ teaspoon salt and a crack of pepper

Prep the salmon by storing the salmon in the fridge skin side up for at 30–60 minutes before cooking. The goal is to dry out the skin which helps make it crispy.

For the wilted kale and mushrooms, remove the stems from the mushrooms and slice the caps thin. Preheat a large non-stick pan just under medium-high heat along with 2 teaspoons of oil for 2 minutes. Add the mushrooms and cook for 5 minutes. Remove the stems from the kale and roughly chop. After 5 minutes, add the onion and red pepper flakes to the pan along with ¼ teaspoon salt and a few cracks of pepper. Cook for another 5 minutes until the veggies are soft, then add the garlic and cook for 1 minute. Add the chopped kale and cook for 5 minutes, then add another ¼ teaspoon salt and the chicken stock or water and cook until the kale has wilted and is soft (about 3–4 minutes). Turn the heat off and add the lemon zest and juice and check for seasoning.

For the tomato salad, add the quartered tomatoes, sliced radishes, and parsley or basil to a bowl. When ready to serve, add the salt, pepper, olive oil, and mix well. Only do this right before serving.

Cook the salmon by preheating a non-stick pan over medium-high heat for 2 minutes. Add 2 teaspoons of oil and wait 30 seconds. Season the skin side of the salmon with a generous amount of salt and place skin side down in the pan. If the oil is not sizzling, remove fish and wait another minute. Season the top side of the salmon with another pinch of salt and allow the salmon to cook undisturbed for 5 minutes. You know the fish is ready to flip when edges on the top turn white and opaque in color. Flip the salmon, turn the heat down just below medium, and allow to cook another 3–4 minutes. If you like your salmon cooked all the way thorough, let it cook 4–5 minutes total on the second side. You can also flip the salmon on the narrower sides and cook for 30 seconds each side. Squeeze the sides of the fish. If it feels firm but still has a little softness, then it is done. Remove from pan and place it skin side up.

Serve the fish with some kale and tomato salad and enjoy!

STORAGE AND REHEATING: Everything will keep in the fridge for three days stored separately. Only the salmon can be frozen for two to three months. Reheat salmon and kale in a 350°F oven for 5–8 minutes or in the microwave.

MACROS

per filet of salmon (makes 3):

223 calories
0 carbs
16 grams of fat
19.3 grams of protein
0 fiber

MACROS

per serving of kale and mushrooms (makes 3):

61 calories
9.2 grams of net carbs
11.6 grams of total carbs
4 grams of fat
4.8 grams of protein
2.3 grams of fiber

MACROS

per serving of tomato salad (makes 3):

52 calories
3.1 grams of net carbs
4.3 grams of total carbs
4.7 grams of fat
1 gram of protein
1.3 grams of fiber

★★★★★

"I just made this recipe tonight and it was super easy and delicious! Thank you for your detailed information about timing and garnishing!" —**Nessa**

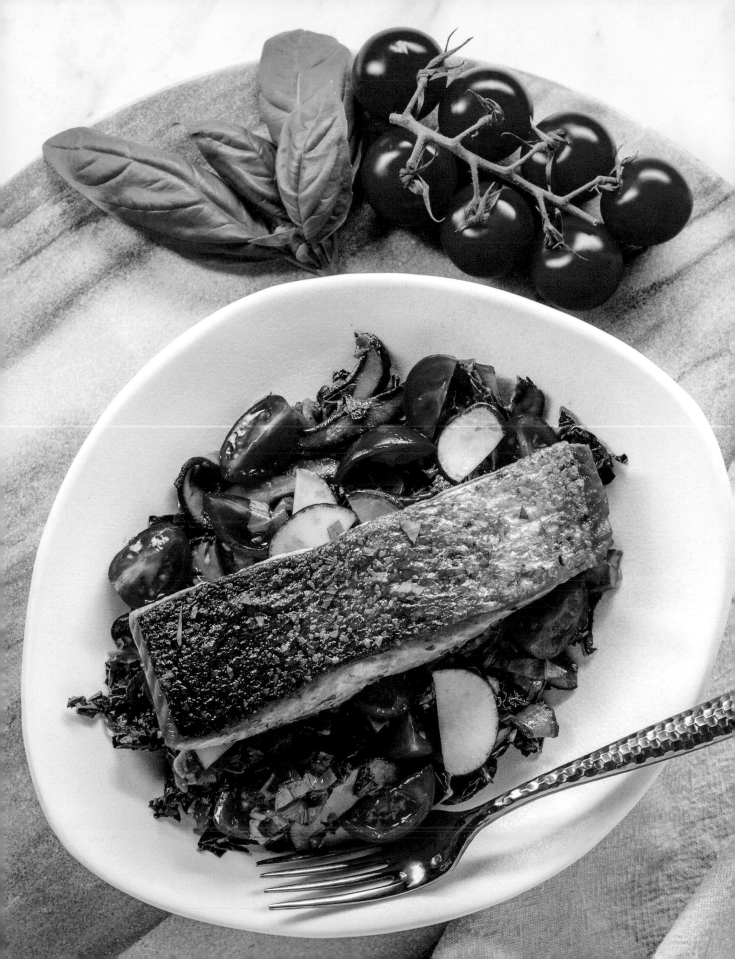

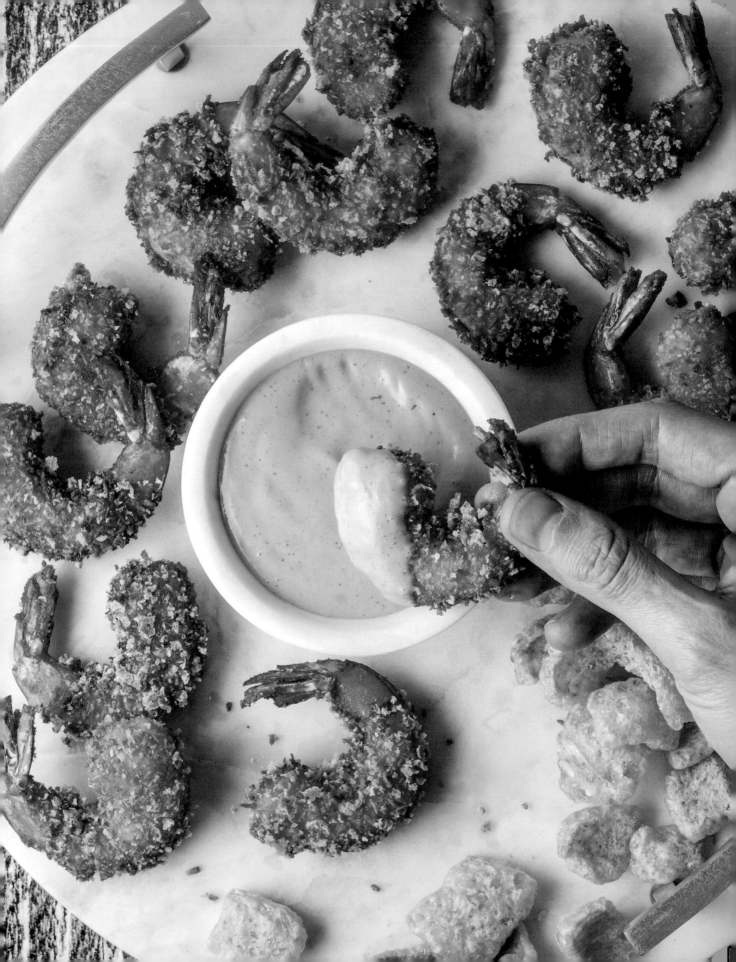

PREP TIME: **10 MINUTES** • COOKING TIME: **10 MINUTES** • MAKES: **4 SERVINGS**

PALEO / WHOLE30

CRISPY COCONUT SHRIMP
WITH CHILI DIPPING SAUCE

Riddle me this food fans: how do you make fried foods crispy when flour and starch are not allowed on the keto diet? Well, it turns out crushed pork rinds and coconut flour do a pretty good job, and, by pretty good, I mean epic! These shrimp are everything you want and more—so crispy and full of flavor.

 To watch the video tutorial for this recipe, search "FlavCity coconut shrimp" on YouTube.

FOR THE SHRIMP:
- ¾ cup coconut flour
- 1 teaspoon garlic powder
- 1 teaspoon onion powder
- 2 eggs, lightly beaten
- ½ cup pork rind crumbs
- ½ cup unsweetened shredded coconut flakes
- 1 pound of large shrimp, peeled and cleaned
- Kosher salt and fresh pepper
- Avocado or expeller pressed sunflower oil

FOR THE DIPPING SAUCE:
- ½ cup full-fat, sugar-free mayonnaise
- Zest and juice of ½ lime
- 1 clove garlic, finely grated
- 2–3 tablespoons sambal oelek or hot sauce
- ¼ teaspoon kosher salt

Prepare the dredge station by adding the coconut flour, onion and garlic powder, ½ teaspoon salt, and a few cracks of pepper to a shallow dish, and mix well. Add the eggs to a small dish/bowl and lightly whisk. Add the pork rinds to a zip-top bag and use a rolling pin to bash them into breadcrumbs the size of panko. Add them to a dish along with the coconut flakes, ¼ teaspoon salt, few cracks of pepper, and mix well.

Season the shrimp with a little pinch of salt on both sides then dredge in the coconut flour, shake off any excess, dredge in the eggs, shake off any excess, dredge in the pork rind and coconut flakes and make sure the shrimp is well covered. Move shrimp to a wire rack set over a sheet tray. Repeat the process with the remaining shrimp.

Pour 2 inches of oil into a frying pan and bring the temperature to 350°F. While the oil is coming to temperature, it's ok that the shrimp sit at room temperature so the coating can firm up. Fry the shrimp in batches for 2–3 minutes on each side or until golden brown. Remove shrimp and place on a clean wire rack; immediately sprinkle with a pinch of salt. Fry the next batch.

Make the sriracha dipping sauce by combining all the ingredients in a small bowl and whisking well. Check for seasoning. You may need more sriracha if you like it spicy.

If using an air fryer to make the coconut shrimp, spray the basket and the shrimp with non-stick and fry for 8 minutes at 390°F, flipping the shrimp halfway.

MACROS

per piece of coconut shrimp:
75 calories
0.9 net carbs
2 grams total carbs
4 grams of fat
3.2 grams of protein
1.6 grams of fiber

MACROS

per tablespoon of sauce:
48 calories
0.11 grams of total & net carbs
2.5 grams of fat
0.08 grams of protein
0 fiber

★★★★★

"I just did the keto version of coconut shrimp in the air fryer; not only did I like them, but my wife thought they were the bomb!" —**Daveo**

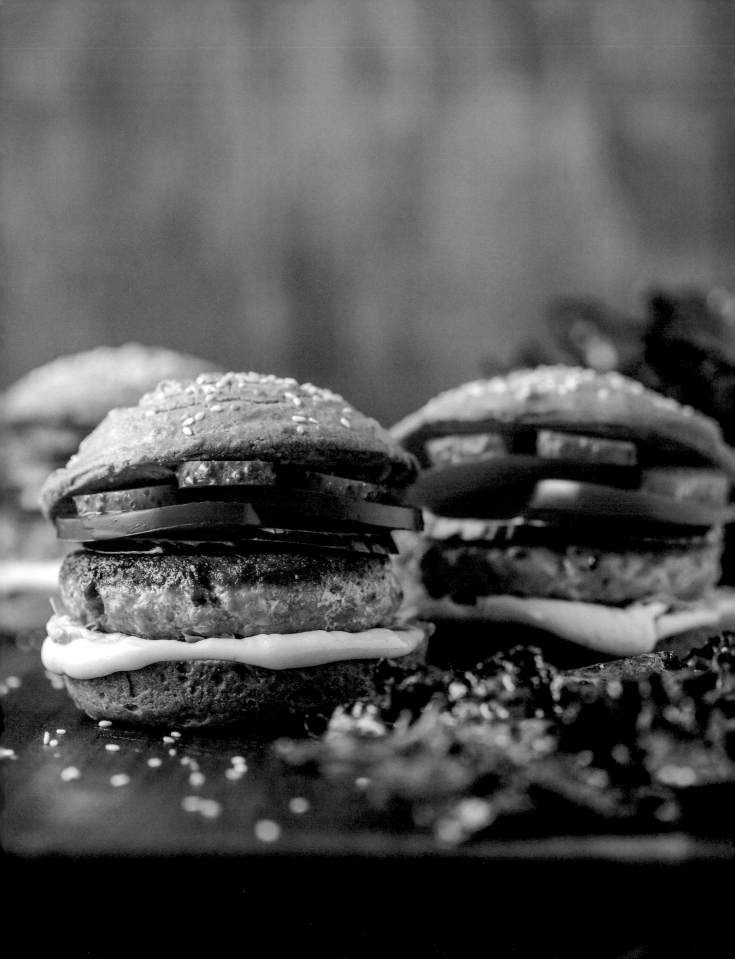

PREP TIME: **30 MINUTES** • COOKING TIME: **45 MINUTES** • MAKES: **5 MEALS**

PALEO

EPIC SALMON BURGERS
AND BBQ KALE CHIPS

When I was a kid, I had a serious obsession with Krunchers BBQ potato chips. Does anyone else remember those? Perhaps that was the reason my doctor was surprised my cholesterol was 360 when I was 7 years old!? These BBQ kale chips are so crispy, smoky, and sweet, and taste just like potato chips if you close your eyes. They go great with my epic salmon burger on fat bread bun. You can't find this a Shake Shack folks!

FOR THE KETO BUNS:
- See recipe for Keto Fat Bread on page 161

Tip | It's best to use an oily salmon such as Atlantic which I buy at Whole Foods. If the salmon is too dense and meaty the texture of the burgers will be off. Make sure to ask your fish monger to remove the skin and cube the salmon since it will save you time.

You Tube | To watch the video tutorial for this recipe, search "FlavCity salmon burger" on YouTube.

FOR THE SALMON BURGERS:
- 2 pounds salmon, skin removed & cut in 1-inch cubes, ask your fish monger to do this
- 2 tablespoons full fat mayonnaise, sugar free
- Zest of 1 lemon
- 1½ teaspoons Dijon or stone-ground mustard
- 1½ teaspoons capers, drained from liquid
- 1 teaspoon smoked paprika
- ½ teaspoon cayenne pepper
- 1 teaspoon kosher salt
- Few cracks of fresh pepper
- 3 tablespoons green onion, finely sliced

FOR THE BBQ KALE CHIPS:
- 2 bunches of black (lacinato) kale
- 1½ teaspoons ancho chili powder
- 1½ teaspoons smoked paprika
- 2 teaspoons brown sugar substitute, like Sukrin Gold
- ½ teaspoon garlic powder
- ½ teaspoon onion powder
- ¼ teaspoon cayenne pepper
- Olive oil
- Kosher salt

To make the salmon burgers, add the ¼ of the cubed salmon to a food processor along with the mayonnaise, lemon zest, mustard, and capers. Puree until the mixture is smooth. Add the remaining salmon cubes and ingredients to the processor. Pulse the processor until the mixture is fairly smooth. Form the salmon mixture into 5 patties. The mixture may be oily and soft, so I like to use an old large mayonnaise or peanut butter lid (3.5 inches wide to make sure the burgers are all the same size. Just make sure to put a layer of plastic wrap over the lid so the burgers pop out easily. Move the formed burgers to the freezer for 15 minutes or the fridge for at least 30 minutes so the salmon firms up.

For the kale chips: Preheat oven to 350°F. Remove the center stalks from the kale, tear leaves into large bite size pieces, and put in a large bowl. Make the BBQ spice rub by combining the ancho chili powder, paprika, brown sugar, garlic powder, onion powder, and cayenne pepper in a small bowl, and mix well. Add 2 tablespoons of olive oil to the kale, ½ teaspoon salt, and all the spice rub. Mix well using your hands and massage the kale to help soften it and thoroughly coat it in the spices, adding more oil if necessary. Taste the kale for seasoning as it may need more cayenne or another pinch of salt.

Working in multiple batches and using two sheet trays, arrange the kale in one single layer and bake for 13-15 minutes. You don't want the kale stacked on top of each other—it should be in one single layer. Kale burns really easily, so make sure to pull it from the oven when the leaves are mostly crispy. It's ok if some look a little wet since they will dry after being removed from the oven. Allow to cool for a couple minutes then use a spatula to scape all the chips off the sheet tray and into a zip-top bag. Repeat with remaining batches.

For the keto buns, see recipe on page 161 to make the batter. You will need to buy a hamburger bun tin that is 1.5 inches deep. I use one from Amazon called "USA pan bakeware mini round cake pans". When the buns come out from the oven, they may have a pointed dome. Rest a ramekin on top and it will push the buns down and make them look good.

To cook the salmon burgers, preheat a large non-stick pan just above medium heat with 2 teaspoons of olive oil. Working in two batches, cook the burgers for 5 minutes or until deep golden brown, flip and repeat. Remove salmon burgers and cook the second batch.

Griddle the buns with some butter in a non-stick pan until golden and serve the burger with toppings of your choice and BBQ kale chips. Enjoy!

STORAGE AND REHEATING: The salmon burgers can stay in the fridge for 3 days or can be frozen for 2-3 months. The kale chips can be stored in a zip-top bag at room temperature for 5 days. The buns can stay in the fridge for 3-4 days or can be frozen for 2-3 months. Thaw and reheat salmon burgers in a 350°F oven for 7-10 minutes, making sure to thaw ahead of time. Or gently reheat salmon patties in a microwave.

MACROS

per salmon patty (makes 5):
323 calories
Less than 0.5 grams net & total carbs
18.6 grams of fat
36.3 grams of protein
0 fiber

MACROS

per serving of kale chips (makes 5):
91 calories
7.4 grams of net carbs
8.7 grams of total carbs
6.2 grams of fat
2.2 grams of protein
1.2 grams of fiber

MACROS

per bun (makes 5):
566 calories
5 grams of net carbs
13.2 grams of total carbs
52.2 grams of fat
10.8 grams of protein
8 grams of fiber

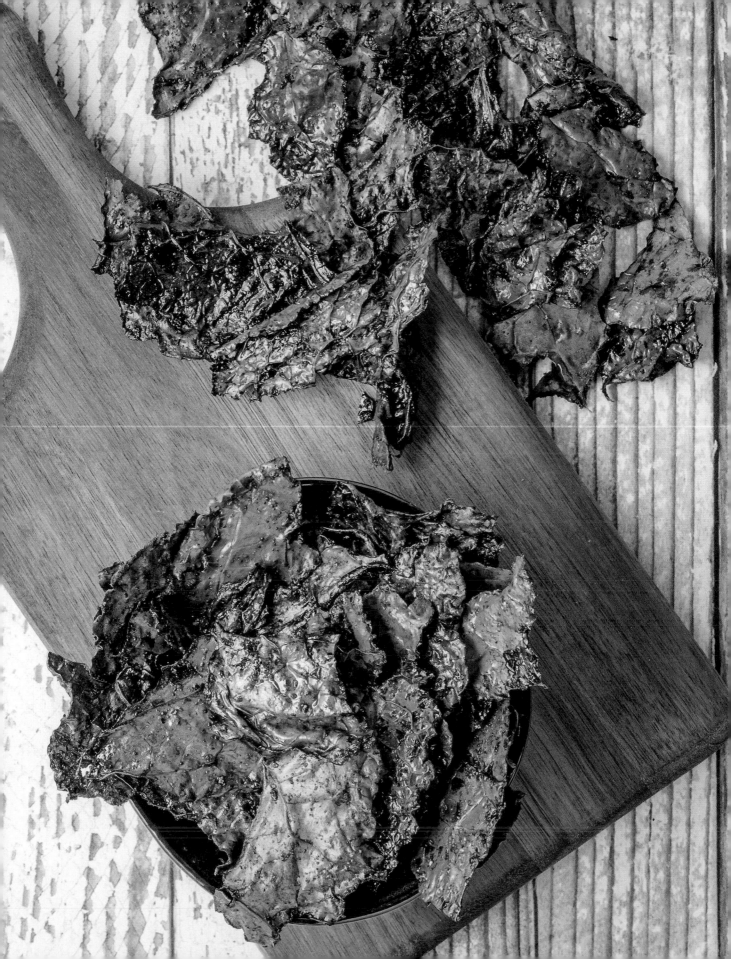

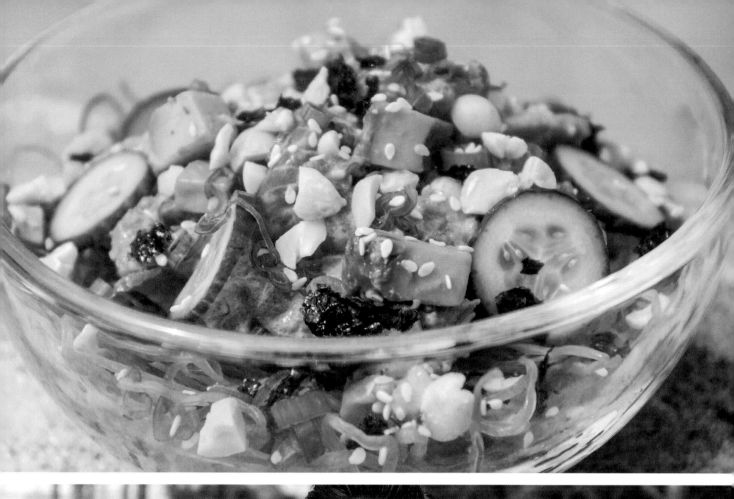

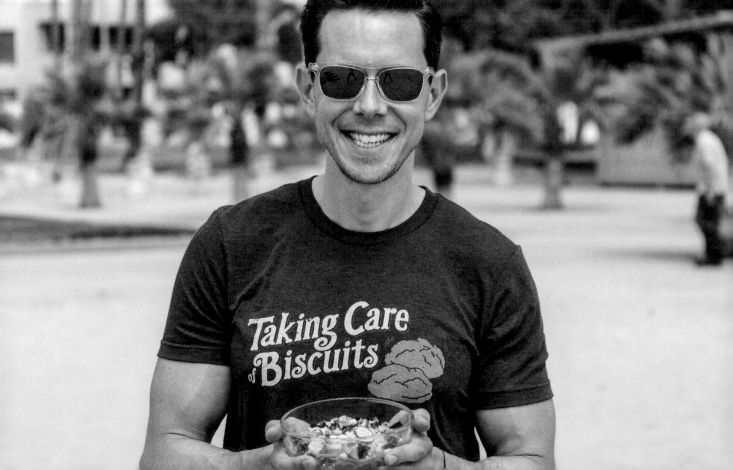

PREP TIME: **10 MINUTES** • COOKING TIME: **5 MINUTES** • MAKES: **2 SERVINGS**

SUMMERTIME SALMON POKE

File this recipe under the category of love-to-eat, hate-to-overpay for it. Poke joints are popping up everywhere, but you can make this no-cook dish at home as long as you have access to sushi-quality salmon from a local fishmonger. I use salmon from Whole Foods. It's very high-quality, farm raised, and fresh enough to eat raw, plus it's so fatty and perfect for poke.

Tip | You can find kelp noodles at Whole Foods. They are a great low-carb substitute for starchy rice in this poke bowls. Alternatively, you can use cooked cauliflower rice.

You | To watch the video tutorial for this recipe, search "FlavCity salmon poke" on YouTube.

FOR THE DRESSING:

- ¼ cup full-fat, sugar-free mayonnaise
- 1–2 tablespoons tamari soy sauce
- 1 teaspoon sambal oelek or sriracha
- ½ teaspoon toasted sesame oil
- Juice of ½ lime
- ½ teaspoon fresh ginger, finely grated using a microplane

FOR THE POKE:

- 8–10 ounces sushi grade salmon, cut in bite-size cubes (have the fishmonger do it)
- 2 tablespoons tamari sauce
- 2 tablespoons green onions, finely sliced
- ¼ cup toasted nuts (macadamia/peanuts), chopped
- 1 small seedless cucumber, finely sliced into rounds
- ½ avocado, diced
- Dried seaweed, for garnish
- Sesame seeds, for garnish
- 1 cup kelp noodles or cooked cauliflower rice
- Lime juice
- ½ teaspoon toasted sesame oil

To make the dressing, add all the ingredients to a small bowl and mix well. If the dressing is a little too thick, add 1–2 tablespoons of water. Check for seasoning. The flavors should really pop, so you might need more tamari or lime juice. In another bowl, toss the salmon cubes with 1 tablespoon of tamari sauce and add enough mayo dressing to coat the salmon. Let marinate in the fridge for 15–30 minutes.

When ready to eat, season the raw kelp noodles or cooked cauliflower rice with 1 tablespoon of tamari, a squeeze of lime juice, and the toasted sesame oil. Add the green onions, toasted nuts, cucumber, and avocado to the salmon mixture. Mix well and serve over a bed of the seasoned kelp noodles or cauliflower rice, garnish with sesame seeds and dried seaweed, and enjoy!

STORAGE: Salmon should not be stored as leftovers and should be enjoyed on the spot.

MACROS

per serving of poke (makes 2):
610 calories
5.15 grams of net carbs
7 grams of total carbs
50 grams of fat
32.2 grams of protein
3 grams of fiber

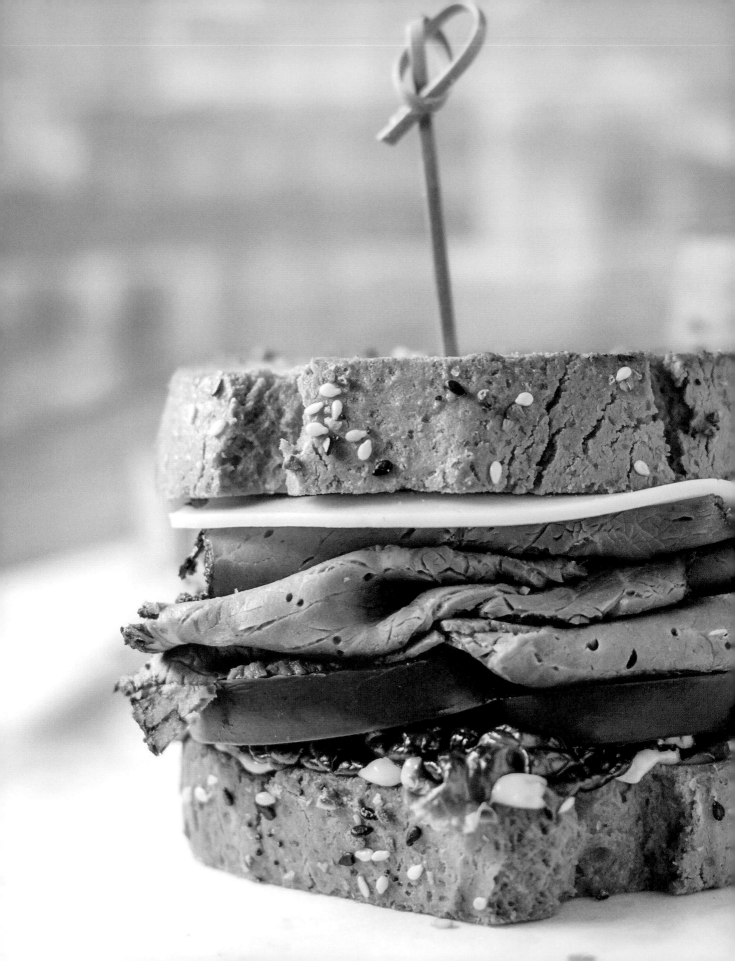

SNACK ATTACK

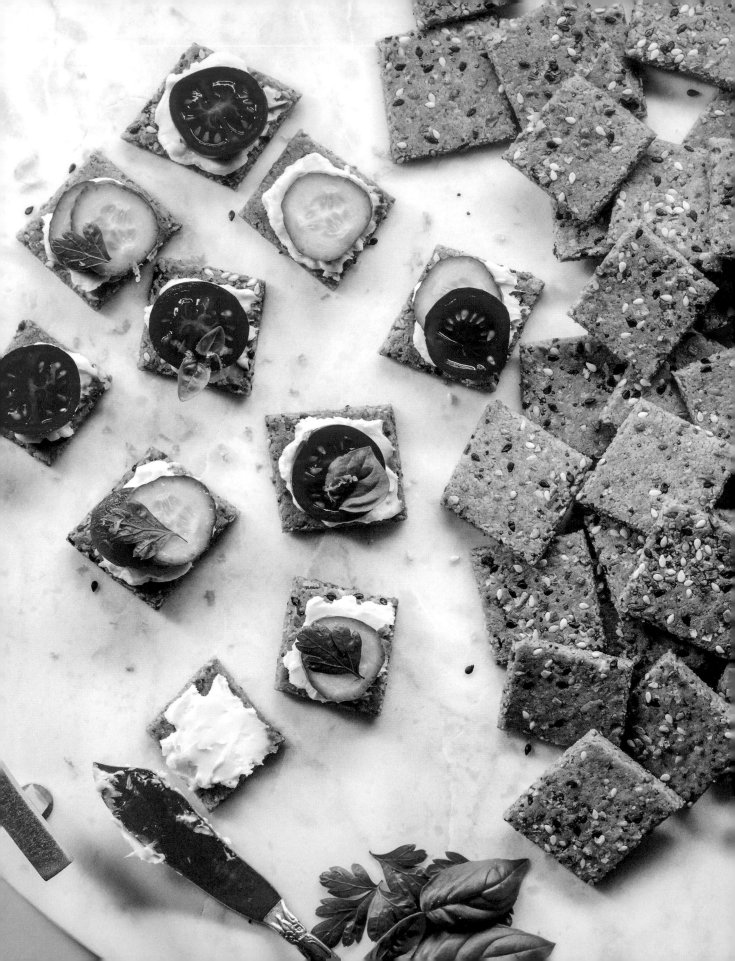

PREP TIME: **20 MINUTES** • COOKING TIME: **45 MINUTES** • MAKES: **ABOUT 66 CRACKERS**

PALEO

DESSI'S EVERYTHING CRACKERS

Dessi used to love almond flour crackers from Simple Mills. The problem is they are not keto and cost twenty dollars per pound! I'm sorry but that's against everything I stand for, so I challenged her to come up with a keto cracker recipe. Thus, we present you with this gem of a snack recipe—both you and your wallet will thank us.

 Tip | You can replace the flax seed egg with two chicken eggs if you don't care about keeping the recipe vegan.

 Tip | If you can't find ground rosemary, finely chop 2 teaspoons of fresh rosemary and use that. Everything bagel seasoning is made of sesame seeds, granulated onion and garlic flakes, and salt. It's sold on Amazon and at Trader Joe's, or you can make it.

You Tube | To watch the video tutorial for this recipe, search "FlavCity keto crackers" on YouTube.

INGREDIENTS:
- 2 tablespoons ground flax meal
- 6 tablespoons water
- 2 cups almond flour, sifted for best results
- ½ cup roasted and unsalted sunflower seeds, ground
- ⅛ teaspoon ground rosemary powder
- ½ teaspoon salt
- 3 cracks of fresh black pepper
- 2 tablespoons extra virgin olive oil
- 1 tablespoon everything bagel seasoning

Preheat oven to 300°F and prepare the vegan flax egg by mixing the flax meal with the water in a small bowl and allowing it to sit at least 15 minutes. Make the sunflower seed flour by grinding ½ cup of seeds in a spice grinder or food processor until it has the texture of flour.

For the dry ingredients, sift the almond flour in a large bowl and add the ground sunflower seeds, ground rosemary, salt, pepper, and combine well using a whisk.

For the wet ingredients, add the olive oil to a small bowl along with the flax eggs, mix well, and add that to the dry ingredients. Mix very well until the dough comes together. This will take a few minutes.

Add a few drops of oil to your hands and spread the dough onto a piece of parchment paper. Place another piece of parchment paper on top and use a rolling pin to flatten the dough into a large rectangle. When the dough is about 80 percent spread, sprinkle the everything bagel seasoning on top and continue to roll out the dough until it takes up the entire width of the parchment paper—the thinner the better.

Use a pizza cutter or a knife to cut the dough into one-inch square cracker shapes. Carefully move the parchment paper with the dough to a sheet tray and bake for 45 minutes or until the crackers are slightly golden, making sure not to burn them.

Remove from oven and allow to cool for at least 15 minutes and enjoy!

STORAGE: Store at room temperature in a zip-top bag for five days.

MACROS

per cracker (makes 66):
26.1 calories
0.35 grams of net carbs
0.79 grams of total carbs
2.3 grams of fat
0.80 grams of protein
0.44 grams of fiber

"Just made them. They are soooooooooooo gooooooood! I can't stop eating them now. Thank you so much for this amazing recipe. You guys are amazing." —**Sikidesi**

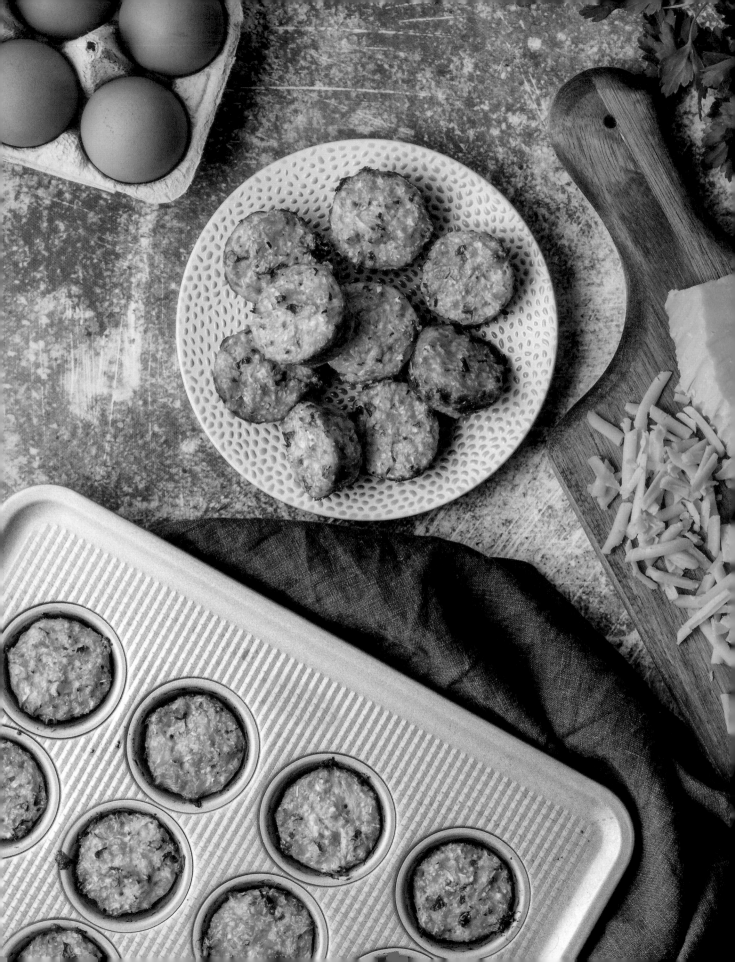

PREP TIME: **15 MINUTES** • COOKING TIME: **20 MINUTES** • MAKES: **24 TOTS**

CHEESY CAULIFLOWER TOTS

I get lots of requests for healthy snacks. It's that time of the day between lunch and dinner when you get a hankering and usually eat something naughty, which is why I created this recipe. The tots are cheesy, golden brown, and low-carb thanks to the cauliflower—exactly what you need when the hunger pains hit.

 This recipe works best with a non-stick mini muffin tin.

 To watch the video tutorial for this recipe, search "FlavCity tots" on YouTube.

INGREDIENTS:

- 1 large head of cauliflower
- 1 cup of shredded cheese, like cheddar or mozzarella (grate it yourself)
- 2 eggs
- 2 tablespoons freshly chopped Italian flat leaf parsley
- ½ teaspoon smoked paprika
- ¼ teaspoon cayenne pepper
- 1 teaspoon olive oil
- Kosher salt and fresh pepper
- Olive or avocado non-stick spray without propellant

Preheat oven to 400°F. Use a box grater or food processor with a grating attachment and grate all the cauliflower, avoiding the stalks. Place the grated cauliflower in a kitchen towel and squeeze as much moisture out as possible. Flex those biceps. The more water you squeeze out, the more golden your tots will be. Place the cauliflower in a large bowl and add all of the remaining ingredients (except the non-stick spray), ¾ teaspoon salt, and few cracks of pepper. Mix well and thoroughly spray the mini muffin tin with the non-stick spray (do this over the sink as to not make as mess everywhere). Use a spoon to add the cauliflower mixture in the tins and pack them so they come all the way to the top. Bake for 25–30 minutes or deep golden brown around the edges. Remove from the oven and let sit for 5 minutes. Then remove from muffin tin and enjoy!

STORAGE AND REHEATING: Tots will keep in the fridge for three days or in the freezer for two to three months. When ready to reheat, place in the microwave or, better yet, reheat in a 350°F oven for 6–8 minutes.

MACROS

per cauliflower tot (makes 24):
32.3 calories
0.87 grams of net carbs
1.3 grams of total carbs
2.3 grams of fat
2 grams of protein
0.46 grams of fiber

★★★★★

"These are SUPER delicious, easy to make, and surprisingly filling. Made a ton and have them in the freezer. Thanks so much for your yummy recipes that are keto friendly. Keep 'em coming!!! You guys are fantastic." —**Christine**

"This recipe is the BOMB! Just made it for my kiddos and they loved it! Thank you so much for creating tots that I can enjoy too!" —**Angela M**

"Wow! These are so so so good. I happen to have ingredients on hand so made them. Slathered them with my keto homemade ketchup and enjoyed. Thanks for sharing." —**Jackie L.**

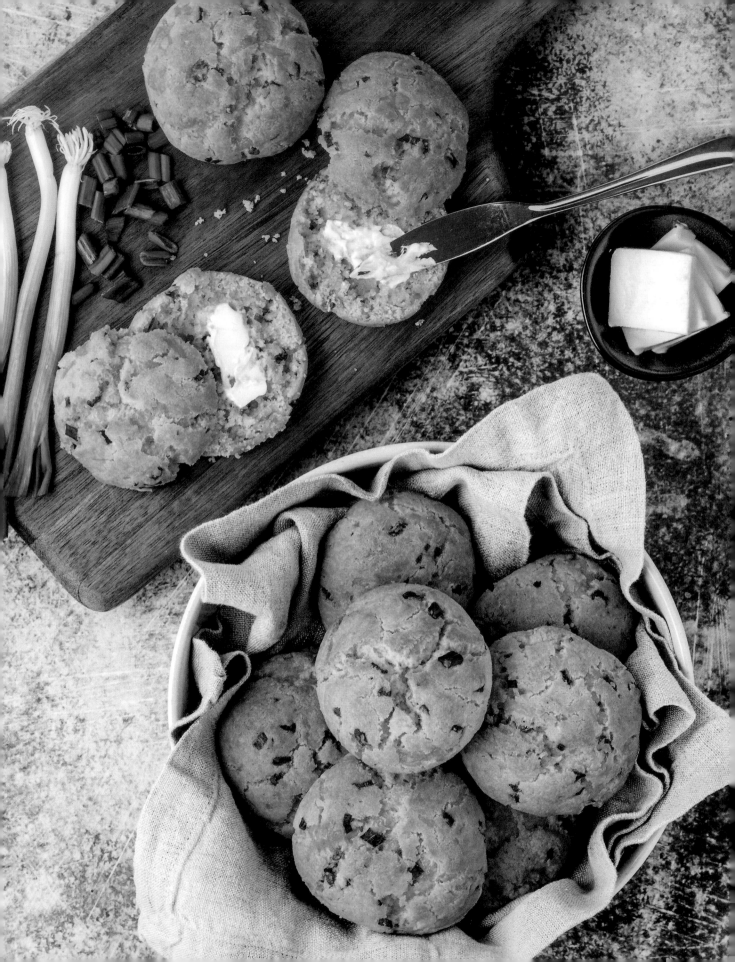

PREP TIME: **20 MINUTES** • COOKING TIME: **20 MINUTES** • MAKES: **10 BISCUITS**

BUTTERY CHEDDAR BISCUITS

I've been to Red Lobster once in my life, and all I remember are those insanely buttery cheddar biscuits. Well, I decided to create a keto version, and let's just say these biscuits are epic...and much healthier.

 Tip | Make sure to use almond flour, not almond meal or coconut flour for this recipe. It's best to buy a block of cheddar cheese and grate it yourself—the pre-grated cheese is coated in anti-caking agents

 | To watch the video tutorial for this recipe, search "FlavCity biscuits" on YouTube.

INGREDIENTS:

- 2 cups almond flour
- 2 teaspoons baking powder
- ½ teaspoon onion powder
- ½ teaspoon garlic powder
- ½ teaspoon kosher salt
- Fresh cracked pepper
- ¼ cup green onions, finely sliced
- 2 eggs, beaten
- ½ cup melted grass-fed butter
- ½ cup cheddar cheese, shredded

Preheat oven to 350°F. In a large bowl, sift in 2 cups of almond flour. If you don't have a sifter, make sure there are no large clumps of flour. Add the baking powder, salt, couple cracks of pepper, onion and garlic powder, and green onions, and mix well. In a small bowl, whisk the eggs, add the melted butter, and whisk well. Pour the wet batter over the dry batter and use a spatula to mix well. Add the shredded cheese and mix until well incorporated. Line a sheet tray with parchment paper and fill a ¼ cup measuring cup about ¾ full of dough. Form the dough into the shape of a large golf ball and place on the parchment paper. Repeat with remaining dough, making sure they are not too close to each other. Bake for 20–23 minutes or until golden brown and remove from oven. Allow to cool for 15 minutes and enjoy!

STORAGE: Biscuits will keep in the fridge for three to four days or can be frozen for two to three months.

MACROS

per biscuit (makes 10):
230 calories
1.8 net grams of carbs
3.6 grams of total carbs
22.4 grams of fat
6.2 grams of protein
1.8 grams of fiber

★★★★★

"That was one of the best biscuits I've had in a long time. I seriously told like ten people about this video. Ah-mazing:)" —**Laura K.**

"Just made the biscuits tonight—they are delicious and light, just like tea biscuits, with our ground beef stew." —**Brenda**

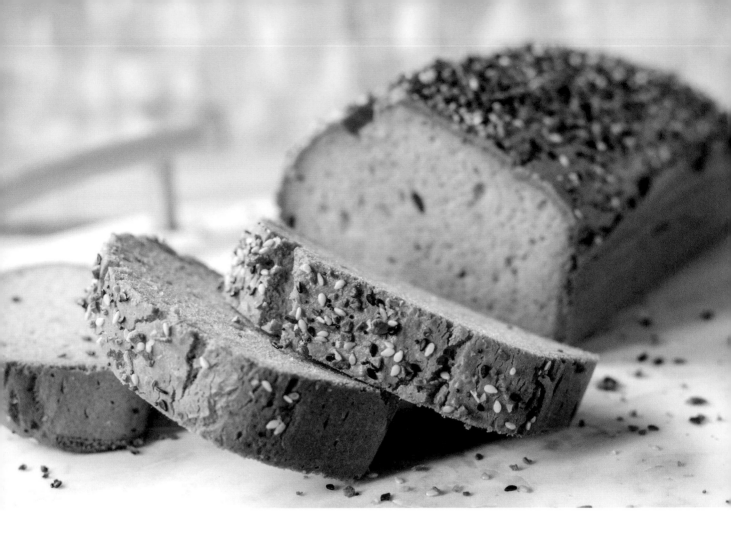

★★★★★

"Just tried this recipe today and it's a winner!! I haven't been able to enjoy bread since I was diagnosed with diabetes about fifteen years ago and this is a game changer. Thank you!!" —**Letty**

"This is the best keto bread I have ever tasted. This is heaven. I finally have toast for the morning and bread for sandwiches. Thank you ever so much. Your channel and website rock!" —**Mick**

"Made this bread yesterday, and it turned out wonderful. So flavorful. I especially love the texture. Now I can add sandwiches back into my diet. Thanks for this recipe." —**Erik and Monica**

"FlavCity knocking it out of the park again! I made this bread today for the first (of what will be many) times and it is amazing! Truly the best keto bread recipe out there. FlavCity has become my and hubby's new fav to watch and get recipes from! Can't wait to try more!" —**Jenny A.**

"I made the keto bread! Wow, I'm so impressed—it's amazing and the everything bagel topping is a nice flavor. I used raw macadamia nuts and mine is a little different color inside than the nice yellow. The flavor is good, but I'm going to use the roasted macadamia nuts next time! You guys are awesome—I love your site! You're my new keto fav!!!!" —**Trease**

PREP TIME: **15 MINUTES** • COOKING TIME: **40 MINUTES** • MAKES: **1 LOAF OF BREAD**   **PALEO**

THE BEST KETO FAT BREAD

Head Notes: If you are looking for keto bread that does not taste eggy and is perfect for making sandwiches, you just found it! The texture of this bread is so great that I've used it to make roast beef sandwiches and even French toast (just don't soak it in the custard for too long).

 Tip

Amazon has the best price on coconut butter (manna)—we like the Nutiva brand. You can use runny almond butter instead of coconut butter, but you can't use coconut oil or cream—it's totally different.

To watch the video tutorial for this recipe, search "FlavCity fat bread" on YouTube.

INGREDIENTS:

- 1 cup macadamia nuts, unsalted and roasted if desired
- 5 good quality eggs
- 1 cup coconut butter (manna)
- ½ teaspoon kosher salt
- 1 teaspoon baking soda
- Zest of ½ lemon
- 1 tablespoon fresh lemon juice
- 1–2 tablespoons everything bagel seasoning

Preheat oven to 350°F and make sure the oven rack is set in the middle of the oven. Add the macadamia nuts to a food processor or a powerful blender and process for about 30 seconds until almost creamy. While the machine is running, add the eggs one at a time, making sure each one has been incorporated into the batter before adding the next one. Turn the machine off and add the coconut butter and salt and process until smooth and creamy. While the machine is off, add the baking soda and lemon zest and juice, and process for 10–15 seconds.

Line the inside of a non-stick 10 x 4.5-inch bread or meatloaf tin with parchment paper. If you don't have parchment paper, rub the inside with coconut or avocado oil or spray with a cooking spray. Pour the batter into the tin and tap it on the counter a couple times. Sprinkle on the everything bagel seasoning and use your fingers to gently press it down into the batter, so it does not fall off. Bake in the oven for 35–38 minutes or until nicely golden brown on top. Remove from oven, allow to sit in tin for 5 minutes, and then lift bread out using the parchment paper and transfer to a cooling rack for 15 minutes.

Slice the bread and enjoy!

STORAGE: Bread will keep for three to four days in the fridge in an airtight container or can be frozen for three months.

MACROS

for a loaf of fat bread:

2830 calories
25 grams of net carbs
66 total carbs
261 grams of fat
40 grams of fiber
54 grams of protein

MACROS

per slice (loaf makes about 14 slices):

202 calories
1.79 grams of net carbs
4.71 total carbs
18.6 grams of fat
2.86 grams of fiber
3.86 grams of protein
2.2 grams of fiber

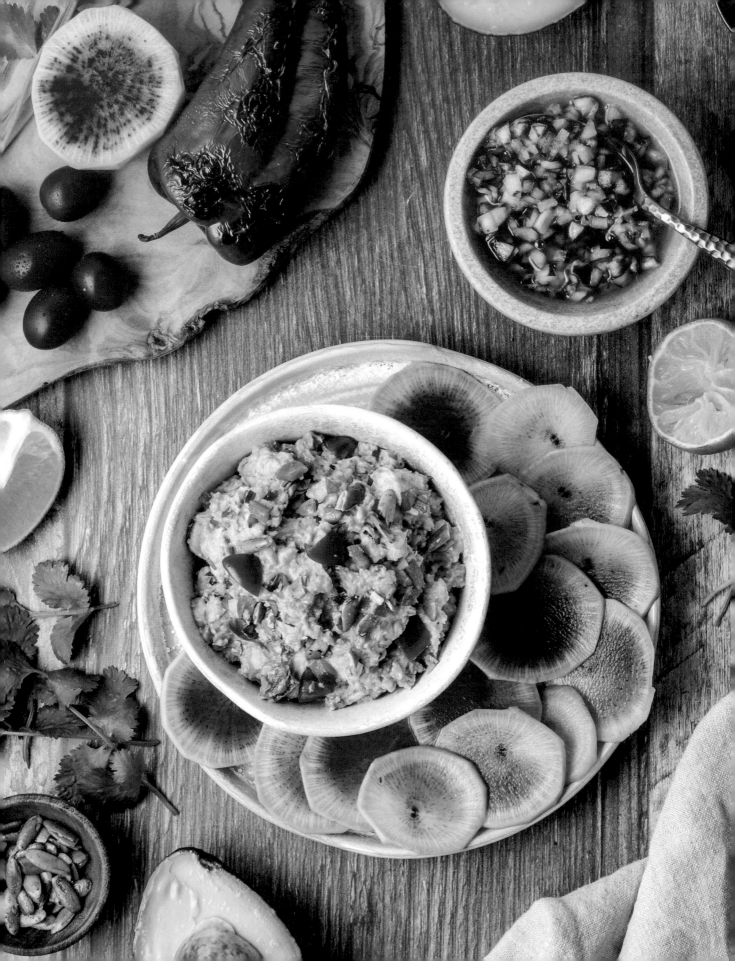

PREP TIME: **10 MINUTES** • COOKING TIME: **10 MINUTES** • MAKES: **4 SERVINGS**

PALEO / WHOLE30

GAME DAY GUACAMOLE

A couple years ago in Mexico City, we discovered the secret to making life-changing guacamole. Never squeeze lime juice directly into the guacamole; it's too acidic and will overpower the delicate flavor of the avocados. Instead, pickle the red onions in lime juice and that's all the acid needed, plus it gets rid of the raw onion flavor. Gracias a todos, Mexico!

 To watch the video tutorial for this recipe, search "FlavCity guacamole" on YouTube.

INGREDIENTS:

- ¼ cup finely chopped red onions
- 1–2 limes
- 1 poblano pepper
- 2 tablespoons pepitas
- ½ teaspoon cumin
- 2 large ripe avocados
- 1 teaspoon extra virgin olive oil
- ¼ cup tomatoes, seeds removed and chopped
- Freshly chopped cilantro or parsley
- Kosher salt

Add the chopped red onions to a small bowl and squeeze over enough lime juice to cover. Allow it to sit for 10–30 minutes. Place the poblano pepper directly on the stovetop burner set to medium-high and char on all sides for about 10 minutes. Remove and place in a bowl and cover with plastic wrap for 5–10 minutes. Then peel away the charred skin, remove the seeds, and finely chop.

Toast the pepitas (Mexican pumpkin seeds) in a non-stick pan with a shot of oil, a pinch of salt, and ½ teaspoon of cumin. Cook over medium heat until golden brown, about 6 minutes. Remove and roughly chop.

Scoop the avocados into a bowl. Add ¼ teaspoon of salt and 1 teaspoon extra virgin olive oil. Next, use a potato masher or large fork to mash to desired consistency. I like it chunky. Add the strained red onions, saving the lime juice, chopped tomatoes, pepitas, poblano pepper, 1–2 teaspoons chopped cilantro, and mix well. Check for seasoning as you may need more salt and reserved lime juice from the red onions.

STORAGE: If not serving immediately, press plastic wrap directly on the surface of the guacamole and keep on the counter for 1 hour or in the fridge overnight.

MACROS

for the entire guacamole:
735 calories
14.5 grams of net carbs
43.2 grams of total carbs
65.2 grams of fat
12.1 grams of protein
28.7 grams of fiber

★★★★★

"OMGoodness!!! You are right! This is the best guac we've ever had! You made me look good, thanks Bobby!" **—Cindy S.**

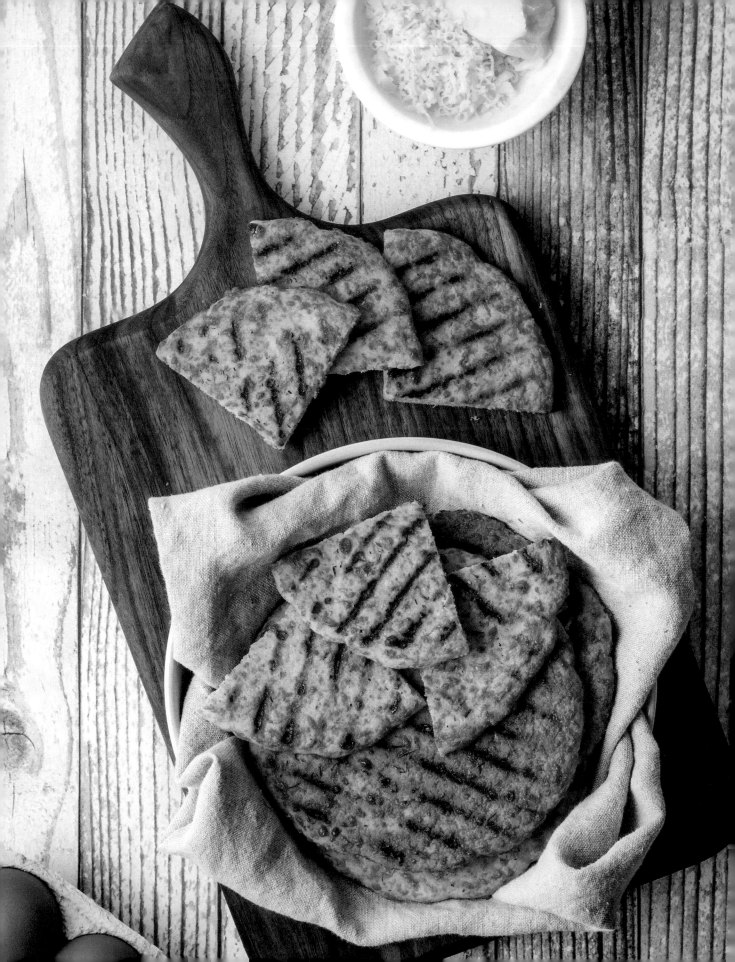

PREP TIME: **15 MINUTES** • COOKING TIME: **15 MINUTES** • MAKES: **5 PITA BREADS**

SOFT AND CHEESY PITA BREAD

Dessi and I went to the Middle East last year and were blown away by the flavors! As soon as we got back, Dessi came up with this keto pita bread recipe so we could fill it with lamb kebabs and creamy tahini sauce. It was a home run!

 Tip | Make sure to buy a block of low moisture mozzarella cheese (Trader Joe's) and grate it on the fine setting of the box grater. Don't buy pre-grated cheese for the pita bread.

 | To watch the video tutorial for this recipe, search "FlavCity pita bread" on YouTube.

INGREDIENTS:

- 2 eggs
- 2 teaspoons baking powder
- ½ teaspoon kosher salt
- 2 cups or 6 ounces by weight of finely shredded full-fat mozzarella cheese
- 1½ cups blanched almond flour
- ½ teaspoon dried thyme

Preheat oven to 400°F. In a large bowl, beat the eggs, add the salt and baking powder, and mix well. Add the finely grated cheese and mix well with a spatula. Add the almond flour and mix well. Put some oil on your hands and continue mixing with your hands. Then separate the dough into five equal balls. Flatten each ball and spread them out on a piece of parchment paper. Next, place another piece of parchment paper on top of the flattened dough. Use a rolling pin to flatten each ball until they are about 5–6 inches in diameter. It's ok if the edges are touching each other. Transfer the dough and bottom piece of parchment to a sheet tray, sprinkle with dried thyme, and bake for 13–15 minutes or until golden brown. Remove from the oven, allow to cool for 5–10 minutes, and enjoy.

STORAGE: Store the pita bread in a zip-top bag in the fridge for three to four days. You can also freeze them for three months.

MACROS

per pita bread (makes 5):
330 calories
4.35 grams of net carbs
7.95 grams of total carbs
27.2 grams of fat
16.8 grams of protein
3.6 grams of fiber

★★★★★

"This flatbread is beyond expectation. I will be using these for other applications: tacos, chalupa, and tostadas just to name a few." —**Adrian E.**

"Bobby, I just made the flatbread and they look, smell, and taste absolutely wonderful." —**Moro G.**

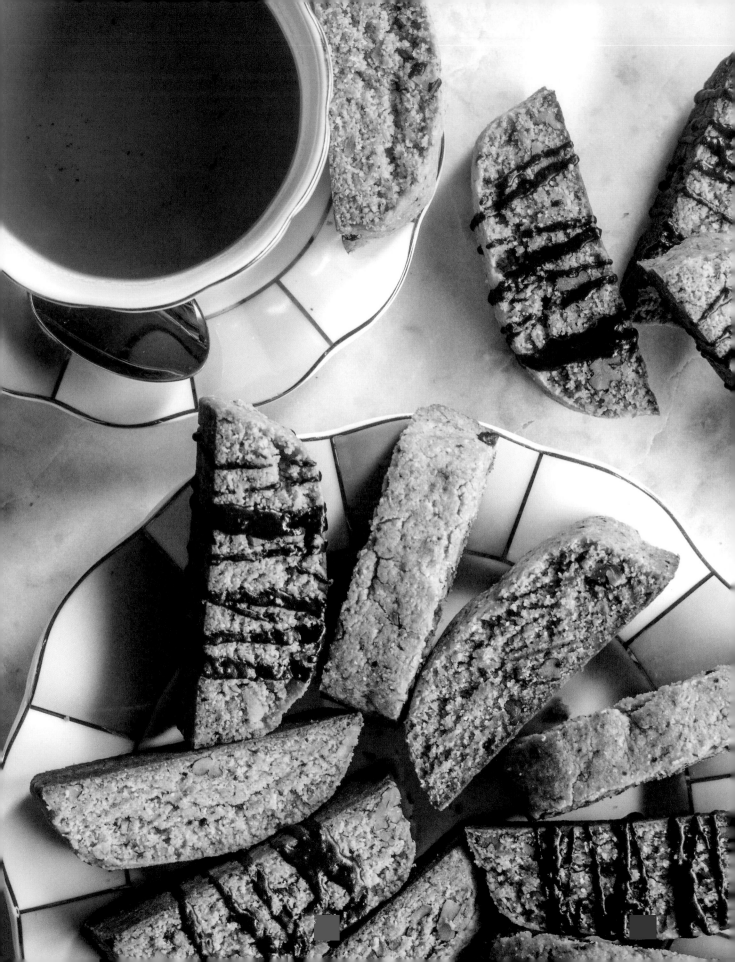

PREP TIME: **20 MINUTES** • COOKING TIME: **1 HOUR** • MAKES: **12 BISCOTTI**

PALEO

NUTTY CHOCOLATE BISCOTTI

We get lots of requests for keto desserts on the FlavCity YouTube channel, and that's where Dessi's expertise comes in handy. These biscotti are just like the real deal. Enjoy them with a spot of tea or our butter coffee (page 35) and your sweet tooth will be satisfied.

 Tip | You can replace the flax seed egg with two chicken eggs for this recipe.

 | To watch the video tutorial for this recipe, search "FlavCity keto biscotti" on YouTube.

FOR THE BISCOTTI:

- 2 tablespoons flaxseed meal (ground flax seeds)
- 6 tablespoons water
- 2 cups almond flour, sifted for best results
- ½ cup sunflower seeds, ground into a flour
- 1 teaspoon baking powder
- ⅓ cup pecans or walnuts, chopped
- Zest of 1 lemon and 1 orange
- 3 tablespoons stevia powder extract
- ¼ cup melted virgin coconut oil or grass-fed butter
- 1 teaspoon pure almond extract

FOR THE CHOCOLATE GLAZE:

- 2 tablespoons finely chopped/shaved bakers' chocolate (100 percent cocoa, no sugar)
- ¼ cup monk fruit sweetener
- 1½ tablespoons virgin coconut oil

Preheat oven to 300°F with the oven rack set in the middle. Prepare the flax egg by mixing the flax meal and water in a small bowl and allow to sit at least 15 minutes so it can thicken.

Sift the almond flour in a large bowl. Use a coffee grinder or food processor to turn the sunflower seeds into flour. To the almond flour, add the ground sunflower seeds, baking powder, lemon and orange zest, and pecans, and mix well with a whisk.

Pour the flax seed egg mixture into a separate bowl and add the stevia powder, almond extract, and coconut oil, and mix well. Add the wet batter on top of the dry batter and mix well until the dough comes together. Use your hands to mix once the dough firms up.

Place a piece of parchment paper on a sheet tray and use your hands and form the dough into a ten-by-three-inch log. You can make the shape wider and shorter if desired. Bake for 35 minutes, then remove from oven and allow to cool down for 15 minutes.

Once cooled, use a sharp knife to cut the log into ¾-inch biscotti pieces and lay them on a cooling rack. Place the cooling rack on the sheet pan and bake for another 25–30 minutes until the biscotti are golden brown and have color around the edges. If you don't have a cooling rack, flip the biscotti halfway to ensure even baking on each side.

For the chocolate glaze, prepare a double boiler or use the microwave to melt the chocolate. Once the chocolate is melted, add the monk fruit sweetener and coconut oil and whisk until the sauce is smooth and creamy. If it is a bit grainy or cools down before drizzling, continue heating until smooth.

Remove biscotti from oven and allow to cool for 10 minutes before drizzling with chocolate sauce. Enjoy!

STORAGE: Chocolate-covered biscotti should be stored in a paper bag at room temperature. Don't place in a sealed zip-top bag because the moister will make them soft. Biscotti will keep for three to four days or can be frozen for three months.

MACROS

per biscotti (makes 12):
210 calories
2.4 grams of net carbs
5.1 grams of total carbs
19.9 grams of fat
5 grams of protein
3 grams of fiber

★★★★★

"This recipe is AWESOME! I used pistachios, and it was so delicious! I'm GF and allergic to eggs, which is no fun when you're Italian! THANK YOU SO MUCH for this recipe!!!!" **—Nina J.**

"Wow, these are delicious. I added a TOUCH of fennel powder to the recipe as that's how my mom used to make them." **—Tuesday**

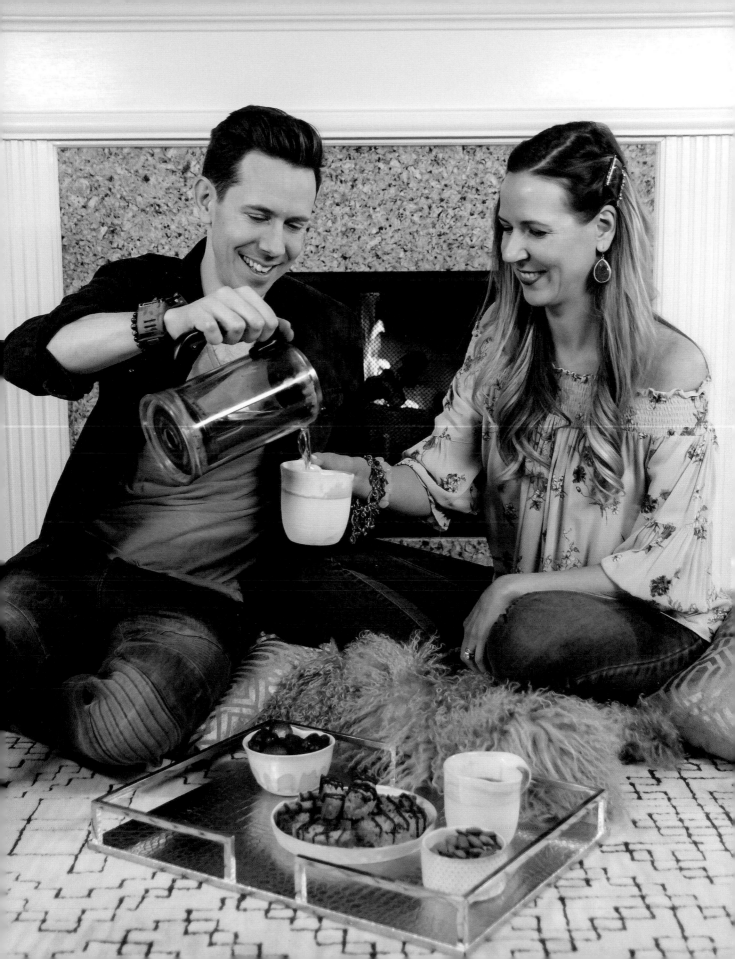

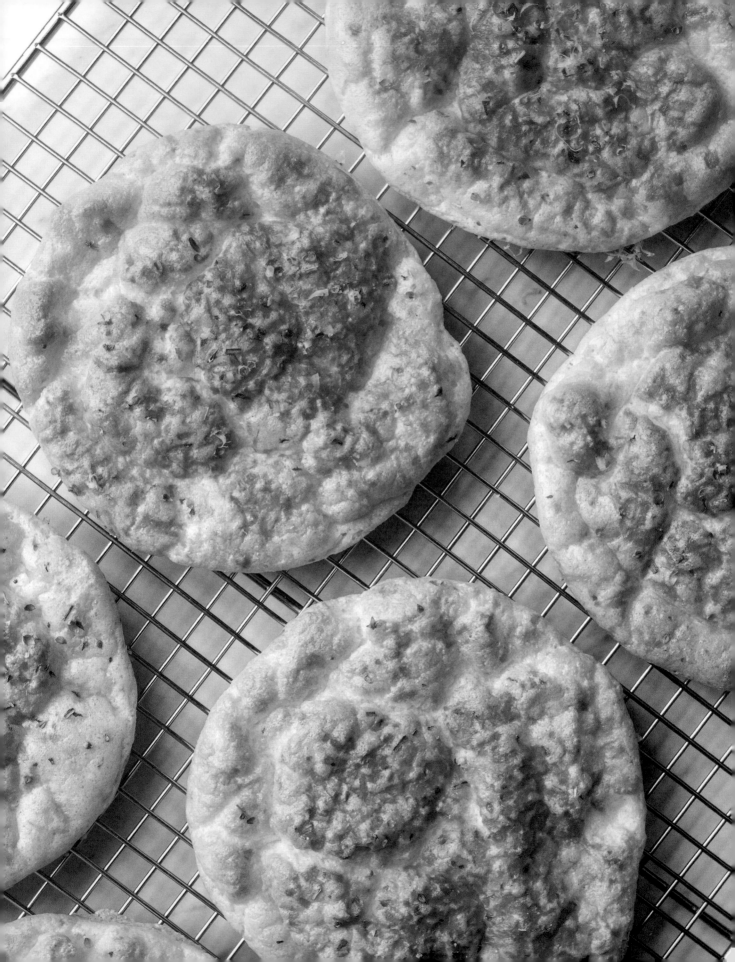

PREP TIME: **20 MINUTES** • COOKING TIME: **30 MINUTES** • MAKES: **8 BREADS**

HERBY CLOUD BREAD

This was my first attempt ever at making keto bread, and I loved it so much that I decided to use it as buns for my roasted chicken salad (see page 61 for recipe). Best lunch ever!

 Tip | The cream cheese for the cloud bread must be at room temperature. Make sure to beat the egg whites to stiff peaks and gently fold in the egg mixture as that is the most important part of the recipe.

 To watch the video tutorial for this recipe, search "FlavCity cloud bread" on YouTube.

INGREDIENTS:

- 6 eggs
- ¼ cup plus 2 tablespoons of room temperature full-fat cream cheese
- ¼ teaspoon cream of tartar
- 1 tablespoon finely grated Parmesan or Pecorino cheese
- ½ teaspoon dried oregano

Preheat oven to 300°F. Make sure the cream cheese is at room temperature or it won't melt into the batter. Carefully crack the eggs, placing the whites in a large bowl and separating the egg yolks in another bowl. If any of the egg yolks breaks into the egg whites, you have to throw them out and start over, so be careful. Add the cream of tartar to the egg whites and use a whisk or hand mixer to beat the egg whites until they reach a stiff peak. If you are not sure what a stiff peak is, watch the video on YouTube. Use the same mixer to combine the egg yolks with the cream cheese and beat until smooth. It's ok if there are little flecks of cream cheese that have not melted. Use a spatula to add half of the egg white mixture to the egg yolks. It is very important that you fold the mixture together and **not stir**— otherwise you will deflate the bubbles. Once the first batch of egg whites is mostly incorporated, add the rest and fold until combined. It's ok if the mixture is not completely smooth: you don't want to overmix the batter.

Place a layer of parchment paper on two sheet trays and use a ½ cup measuring cup to scoop the batter on to the parchment paper. Try to make the shape the size of a bun and use a spoon to make it even. The batter will spread a little, so make sure not to make them too thin or wide. Grate a little bit of cheese and sprinkle a little of the oregano on the top of the buns. Bake in the oven for 27–30 minutes or until deep golden brown in color. Remove from oven and allow to cool.

STORAGE AND REHEATING: The cloud bread should be cooled and stored in a zip-top bag in the fridge for four to five days or can be frozen and reheated in a warm oven.

MACROS | **per cloud bread (makes 8):**
93 calories
0.74 grams of net and total carbs
9.6 grams of fat
5.5 grams of protein
0 fiber

★★★★★

"I have made cloud bread, but this recipe is by far the best. Adding the spice and cheese is amazing. Thank you 'flavor king'!" —**Darlene J.**

"First time making the cloud bread and it's amazing! Will definitely make it more often." —**Tonya**

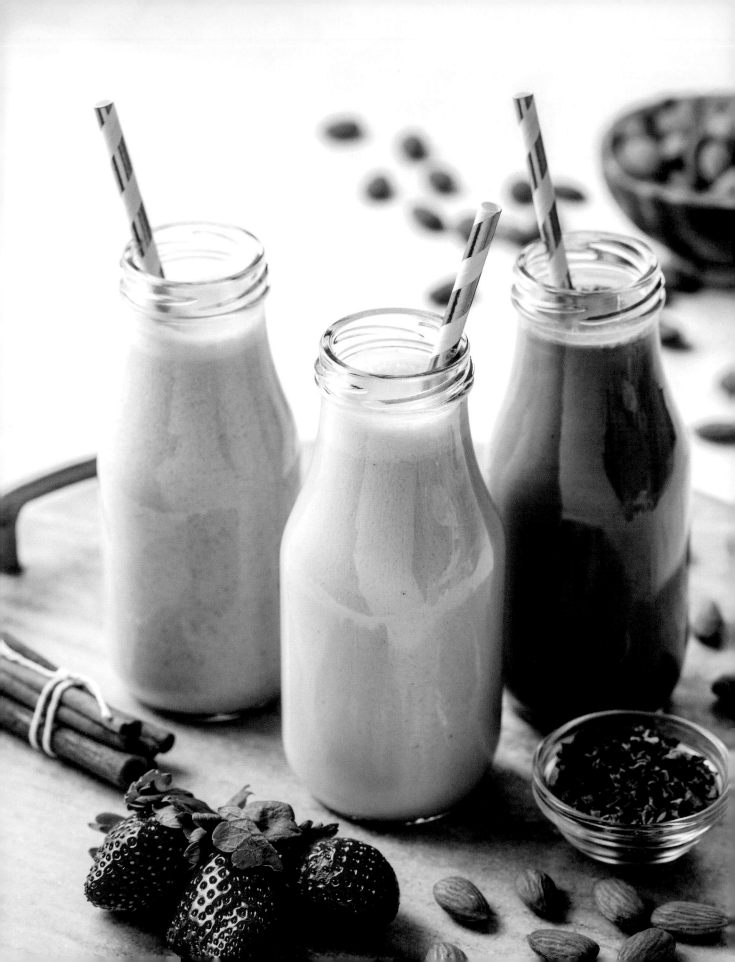

PREP TIME: **6–12 HOURS** • COOKING TIME: **10 MINUTES** • MAKES: **5½ CUPS OF ALMOND MILK**

PALEO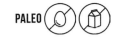

HOMEMADE ALMOND MILK—THREE WAYS

If you think the almond milk you buy at the store is good, then you ain't seen nothing yet! Turns out the store-bought almond milk is mostly water and emulsifiers: all filler and no thriller. Dessi's homemade version is the real deal, and the flavor is so rich and creamy.

 Tip

To make the almond milk sweet and creamy, it is best to blanch the soaked almonds in boiling water for 1 minute and then peel the skins off. I know this is a bit of work, but the skin can give a slightly bitter flavor.

To watch the video tutorial for this recipe, search "FlavCity almond milk" on YouTube.

FOR THE ALMOND MILK BASE:

- 1½ cup almonds
- 44 ounces filtered water
- 30–35 drops of stevia
- 1 teaspoon vanilla paste or extract

FOR THE VANILLA CINNAMON MILK:

- 5½ cups (44 oz) of almond milk
- 1½ teaspoon of cinnamon

FOR THE STRAWBERRY MILK:

- 5½ cups (44 oz) of almond milk
- 1½ cups of cleaned and chopped organic strawberries

FOR THE CHOCOLATE MILK:

- 5 ½ cups (44 oz) of almond milk
- 3 tablespoons of unsweetened cocoa powder

Make base by soaking 1½ cups almonds with enough water to cover by 1 inch. Store in fridge and allow to soak for at least 6 hours, but preferably overnight. Drain the almonds, boil them for 1 minute, and then run them under cold water. Peel the brown skin off and throw it away. Add peeled almonds to the blender along with 44 ounces of filtered water and blend on high for 2 minutes. Pour mixture into a nut milk bag, set in a large bowl, and strain. Throw away the solids remaining in the bag and add 30 drops of stevia to the liquid along with the vanilla paste/extract. Whisk well and check for seasoning as you may need more stevia or vanilla. Store milk in fridge the flavor and texture improve greatly after 8 hours.

For the vanilla cinnamon almond milk, add cinnamon to the base recipe and whisk very well.

For the strawberry almond milk, add the strawberries to a blender with the base recipe and blend on high for 30 seconds. Use the nut milk bag to strain the mixture into a large bowl for a silky texture.

For the chocolate milk, add the cocoa powder to the blender with the base recipe and blend on high for 30 seconds.

STORAGE: Milk will keep in the fridge for three to four days.

MACROS

per 8-ounce cup of almond milk:

30 calories
0.3 grams of net carbs
    (3.3 grams for strawberry)
1 gram of total carbs
    (4.1 grams for strawberry)
2.5 grams of fat
1 gram of protein
0.7 grams of fiber

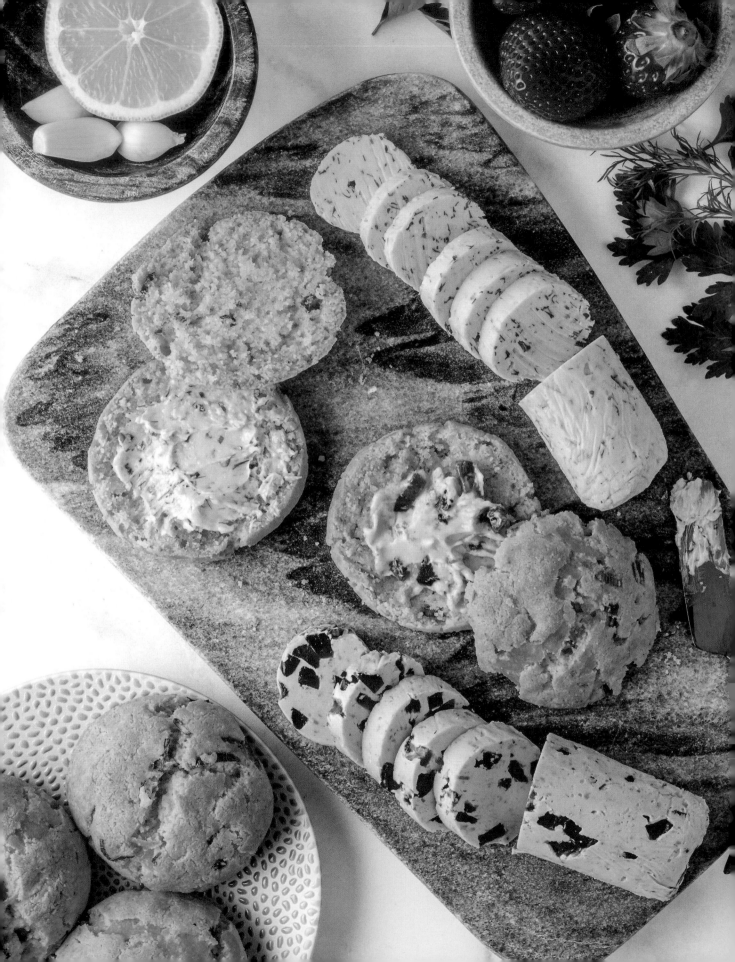

PREP TIME: **5 MINUTES** • COOKING TIME: **5 MINUTES** • MAKES: **2 STICKS OF BUTTER**

STRAWBERRY AND CITRUS HERB BUTTERS

I love flavor bombs! They usually come in the form of pantry items or freezer staples and add massive flavor to anything you are cooking. Soy sauce and tomato paste are the ones people usually think of, but, once you make these flavored butters, they will be your new favorite culinary weapons.

FOR THE STRAWBERRY BUTTER:

- 1 stick unsalted grass-fed butter, room temperature
- ¼ cup strawberries, finely cubed
- 2–3 liquid stevia drops
- Zest of ½ orange
- ¼ teaspoon kosher salt

FOR THE CITRUS HERB BUTTER:

- 1 stick unsalted grass-fed butter, room temperature
- Zest of one lemon
- 1 teaspoon fresh parsley, finely chopped
- 1 teaspoon dill, finely chopped
- 1 clove garlic, finely grated
- Kosher salt and fresh pepper

For the strawberry butter, add everything to a medium-sized bowl and use a hand mixer to beat well. You can use a spatula, but a hand mixer is best. Taste some of the butter—you may need more stevia. Tear off a large piece of plastic wrap, scoop the butter in the middle, and use the wrap to roll the butter into a log. Securely tighten the butter and keep in the fridge for three to four days or freeze for two months. Use this butter on a on a slice of Keto Fat Bread (page 161) or my Buttery Cheddar Buscuits on page 159.

For the herb butter, add all ingredients to a medium-sized bowl and beat well with a hand mixer. You can also use a spatula. Tear off a large piece of plastic wrap, scoop the butter in the middle, and use the wrap to roll the butter into a log. Securely tighten the butter and keep in the fridge for two weeks or freeze for two months. Feel free to use this butter on any chicken, pork, or beef dish in the book. You can even make scrambled eggs with it, brilliant!

MACROS

for all the strawberry butter:
974 calories
2.3 grams of net carbs
3 grams of total carbs
112 grams of at
1 gram of protein
0 fiber

MACROS

for all the herb butter:
968 calories
1.1 grams of net carbs
1.3 grams of total carbs
112 grams of fat
1 gram of protein
0 fiber

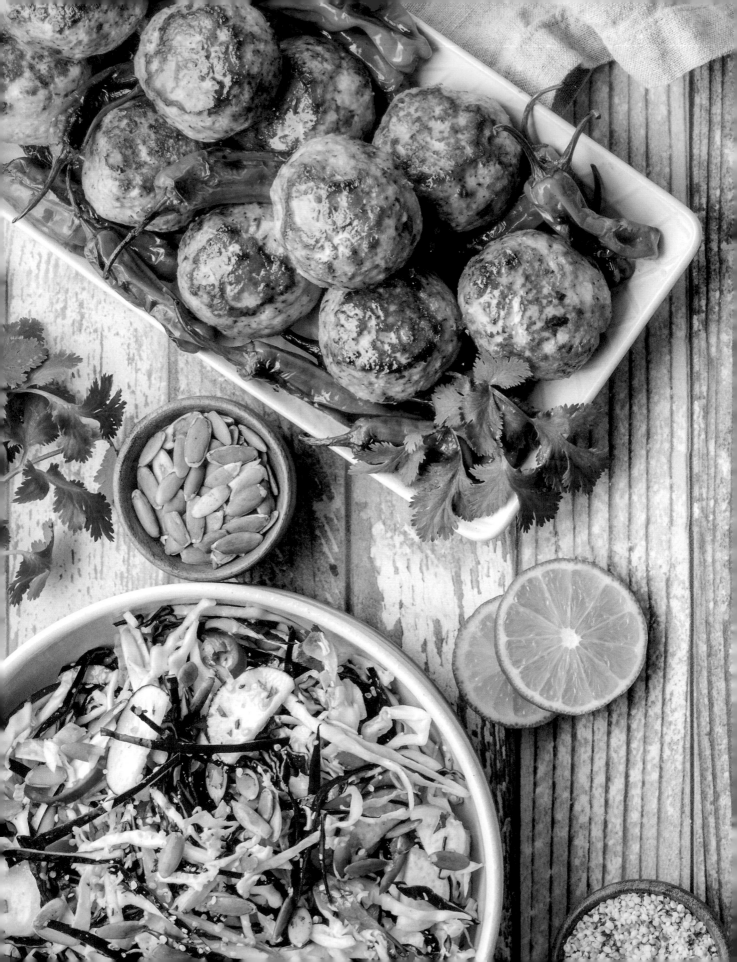

TURKEY— IT'S NOT JUST FOR THANKSGIVING!

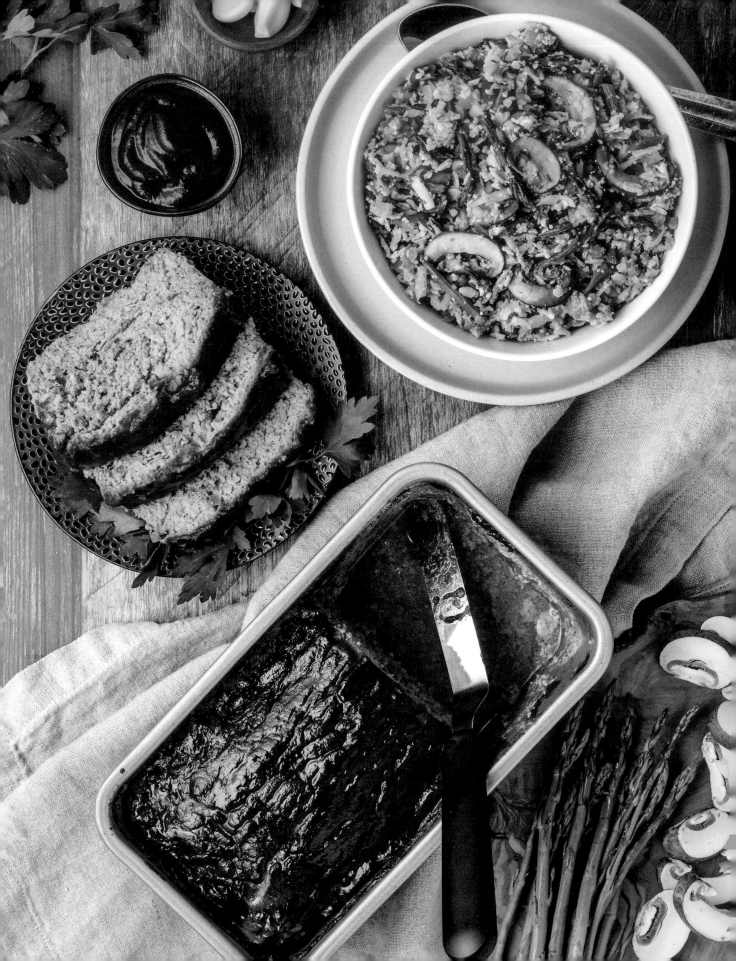

PREP TIME: **20 MINUTES** • COOKING TIME: **60 MINUTES** • MAKES: **5 MEALS**

PALEO

TURKEY MEATLOAF
AND CAULIFLOWER RICE PILAF

No starchy filler needed for this veggie-loaded turkey meatloaf with a classic (sugar-free) ketchup glaze. I've been told many kids have been fooled by this meal, thinking they were eating beefy meatloaf and rice! And, of course, their parents didn't tell them any different!

Tip

It's best to bake the meatloaf in a loaf pan. The ground turkey mixture is loose; if you try to bake it free-form on a sheet tray it will spread out and lose its form.

FOR THE MEATLOAF:

- ½ onion, finely chopped
- 2 stalks of celery, diced
- 1 green bell pepper, diced
- 1 teaspoon dried thyme
- 3 cloves of garlic, minced
- 2 pounds ground turkey thighs
- 1 egg
- 1 tablespoon Worcestershire sauce
- ½ cup plus 3 tablespoons of sugar-free ketchup (to make your own, watch my recipe on YouTube)
- 1 tablespoon fresh Italian parsley, chopped
- Olive oil
- Kosher salt and fresh pepper

FOR THE CAULIFLOWER RICE PILAF:

- 1 large head of cauliflower
- ½ onion, chopped
- 8 ounces cremini or baby bella mushrooms, sliced
- ½ pound asparagus, sliced
- 1 medium-sized zucchini, chopped
- ½ teaspoon dried thyme
- 2 cloves of garlic, minced
- Zest of 1 lemon
- 2 teaspoons fresh chives, chopped
- 2 teaspoons parsley, chopped
- Olive oil
- Kosher salt and fresh pepper

For the meatloaf, preheat oven to 350°F. Preheat a large pan over medium heat with 1 tablespoon of olive oil for 2 minutes. Add the onions, celery, green peppers, dried thyme, ½ teaspoon salt, and a couple crack of black pepper. Cook for 10 minutes, stirring a few times. Add the minced garlic and cook for another 6 minutes or until the veggies have wilted down. Check for seasoning as you will most likely need to add a little more salt. Set the pan aside and allow to cool for 5–10 minutes. Meanwhile, in a large bowl, add the ground turkey, egg, Worcestershire sauce, 3 tablespoons of ketchup, 1 tablespoon of parsley, 1 teaspoon salt, and a few cracks of pepper. Once the veggie mixture has cooled down, add all of it to the bowl with the turkey and mix until just incorporated.

Pour the turkey mixture into a meatloaf pan, pack it well, and cover with your desired amount of ketchup. Place the loaf pan on a sheet tray and bake for roughly 45 minutes, or until the internal temperature in the middle of the loaf is 155°F.

Make the cauliflower rice pilaf by cutting the head of cauliflower into four smaller pieces and grating it on the largest part of a box grater (trying not to grate too much of the stalk) and setting aside. Preheat a large pan over medium heat with 1 tablespoon of olive oil for 2 minutes. Add the onions, mushrooms, asparagus, zucchini, dried thyme, ½ teaspoon salt, and few cracks of pepper. Cook for 10 minutes, stirring a few times. Add the garlic and cook another 3 minutes. Add the grated cauliflower along with ¼ teaspoon of salt, mix well, and place a lid or a sheet tray over the top of the pan and let it steam for 4 minutes. Make sure not to overcook the cauliflower rice; you want it to have a bite. Turn the heat off and add the lemon zest, parsley, and chives, and check for seasoning. You may need a little more salt or a squeeze of lemon juice. Mix well and set aside.

Once the meatloaf is done, allow it to cool for 20 minutes before you cut it; otherwise, it will fall apart. Serve the meatloaf with the pilaf and enjoy!

STORAGE AND REHEATING: The meatloaf and cauliflower rice pilaf will keep in the fridge for five days, or you can freeze the meatloaf for two to three months (not the pilaf). Reheat in a 350°F oven for 7–10 minutes. If you are using a microwave, take the lid off, cover the container with a wet paper towel—this will keep the meatloaf moist.

Keto Meal Prep

MACROS

per serving of meatloaf (makes 5):

325 calories

5.1 grams of net carbs

7 grams of total carbs

21.4 grams of fat

24.4 grams of protein

1.3 grams of fiber

MACROS

per serving of pilaf (makes 5):

76 calories

7.6 grams of net carbs

12.4 grams of total carbs

2.6 grams of fat

4.9 grams of protein

4.2 grams of fiber

 "To watch the video tutorial for this recipe, search "FlavCity turkey meatloaf" on YouTube."

★★★★★

"This is the Bomb! I just tried it; it's so tasty and quite filling even though it was a small serving. Love love love this! You're the best! I love your channel." **—Miz T**

"Talk about heaven on your taste buds!! This meatloaf was the best tasting thing ever!!! Thank you so much! I can't wait to try other recipes. As long as they are as good as that meatloaf, I'll be a happy camper on this lifestyle journey." **—Rashadda W.**

PREP TIME: **25 MINUTES** • COOKING TIME: **30 MINUTES** • MAKES: **5 MEALS**   **PALEO**

MEXICAN TURKEY MEATBALLS
WITH CRUNCHY CABBAGE SALAD

I feel like ground turkey thighs don't get enough love; they are so juicy and make the perfect meatballs, especially when loaded with crunchy pepitas and spices. Eating shishito peppers is like playing culinary Russian roulette. One out of ten is spicy. You just never know when it's going to hit you!

FOR THE SHISHITO PEPPERS:
- 12 ounces shishito peppers
- 1 lime
- Kosher salt and fresh pepper
- Avocado oil

FOR THE MEATBALLS:
- 2 pounds ground turkey thigh
- 1½ teaspoons cumin
- 1½ teaspoons ancho chili powder
- ½ teaspoon cayenne pepper
- ¾ teaspoon dried thyme
- 3 tablespoons pepita seeds, roughly chopped
- 1 tablespoon fresh cilantro or parsley, chopped
- Kosher salt and fresh pepper
- Avocado or olive oil

FOR THE SALAD:
- ½ medium-sized head of red cabbage
- ½ medium-sized head of green cabbage
- ¼ cup hemp hearts
- ¼ cup pepitas, toasted and chopped
- 3 tablespoons cilantro, chopped
- 1 red finger chili, finely sliced
- ⅓ cup radishes, thinly sliced
- Kosher salt and fresh pepper
- ¼ cup extra virgin olive oil
- Juice of 1 large lime
- ½ teaspoon ground cumin
- 3 drops liquid stevia
- 1 clove garlic, finely grated

Tip You can find shishito peppers at Trader Joe's or Whole Foods. You can save time by buying a large bag of cabbage slaw mix for this recipe.

To watch a similar video tutorial for this recipe, search "FlavCity Mexican meatballs" on YouTube.

For the meatballs, add the ground turkey to a large bowl along with the ancho chili, cumin, cayenne, thyme, pepitas, cilantro, 1½ teaspoons salt, and a few cracks of pepper. Mix until just combined and then dip your hands into water (which prevents the meat from sticking to your hands) and form meatballs that are slightly larger than a golf ball. This recipe should make fifteen balls. Store formed meatballs in the fridge for at least 20 minutes, so they can firm up. Preheat oven to 350°F.

Preheat a large non-stick pan over medium-high heat for 2 minutes. Add 1 tablespoon of oil to the pan and wait 30 seconds before adding half of the meatballs to the pan, making sure not to overcrowd the pan. Cook on one side for 1–2 minutes or until golden brown, flip, and repeat. Remove meatballs from pan and place on a sheet tray. Repeat with remaining meatballs. Bake meatballs in the oven for 15 minutes. If you are not sure the meatballs are cooked through, cut one in half. Ground turkey can overcook and become dry very quickly, so make sure to check the meatballs after 15 minutes.

Make the shishito peppers while the meatballs are in the oven. Preheat the same pan just below high heat. Add 2 teaspoons of oil to the pan along with all the shishito peppers. Cook for 7–10 minutes or until charred and blistered on all sides, stirring often. Turn the heat off and season with a pinch of salt and the juice of half a lime and mix well. Remove peppers from pan and set aside.

Make the salad by slicing the red and green cabbage very thin and adding to a large bowl. Add the hemp hearts, pepitas, cilantro, red chili, radishes, pinch of salt, and a few cracks of pepper. To make the dressing, add the lime juice, cumin, stevia, grated garlic, ¼ teaspoon salt, and a few cracks of pepper to a bowl. While whisking, add the olive oil and mix well. Check for seasoning—the dressing should be on the acidic side, so you may need more lime juice and perhaps more cumin. Only dress the salad right before enjoying or 3 hours before as it won't get soft and wilted if taking to work.

Serve the meatballs with the peppers and salad and enjoy!

STORAGE AND REHEATING: Everything will keep in the fridge for five days. Only the meatballs can be frozen for two to three months. Reheat the peppers and meatballs in a 350°F oven for 7–10 minutes or gently reheat in a microwave, covered with a wet paper towel.

MACROS

per serving of meatballs (makes 5):
310 calories
1 gram of net carbs
1.4 grams of total carbs
24.1 grams of fat
23.9 grams of protein
0.4 grams of fiber

MACROS

per serving of salad (makes 5):
216 calories
6.6 grams of net carbs
11.1 grams of total carbs
18.2 grams of fat
6.5 grams of protein
4.5 grams of fiber

MACROS

per serving of peppers (makes 5):
28 calories
0.8 grams of net carbs
2.4 grams of total carbs
2 grams of fat
1.6 grams of protein
1.4 grams of fiber

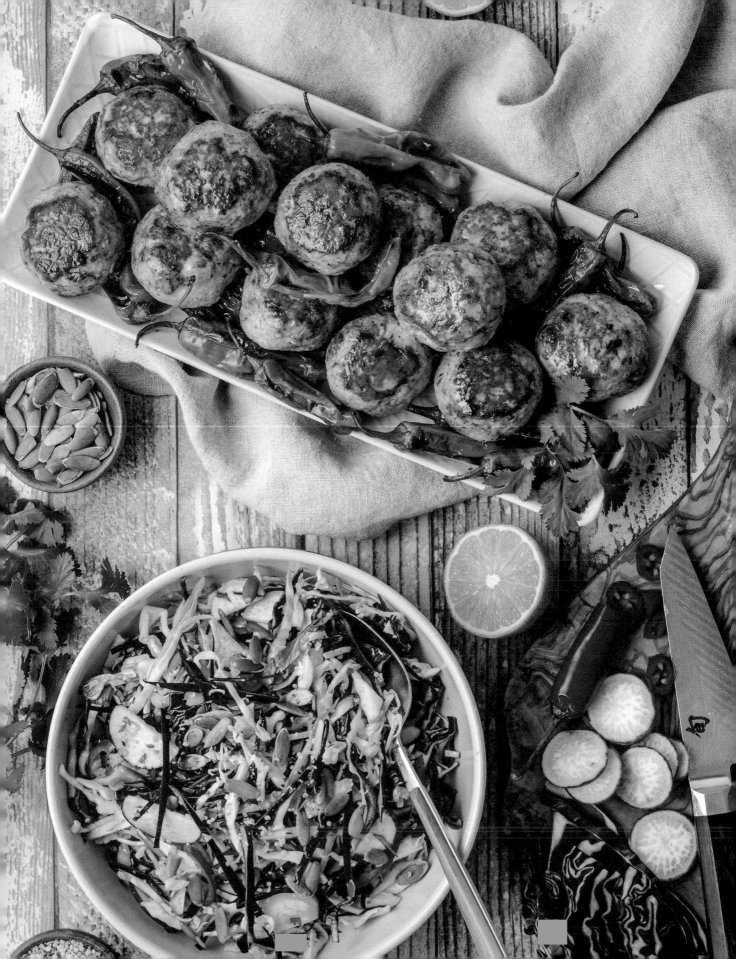

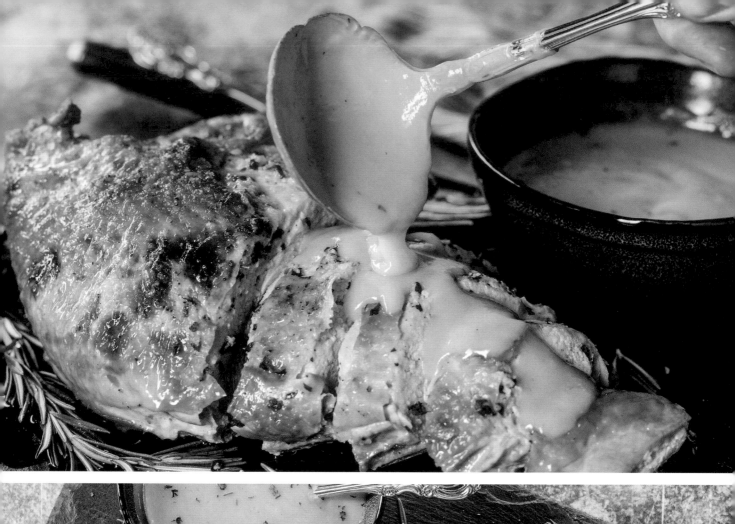

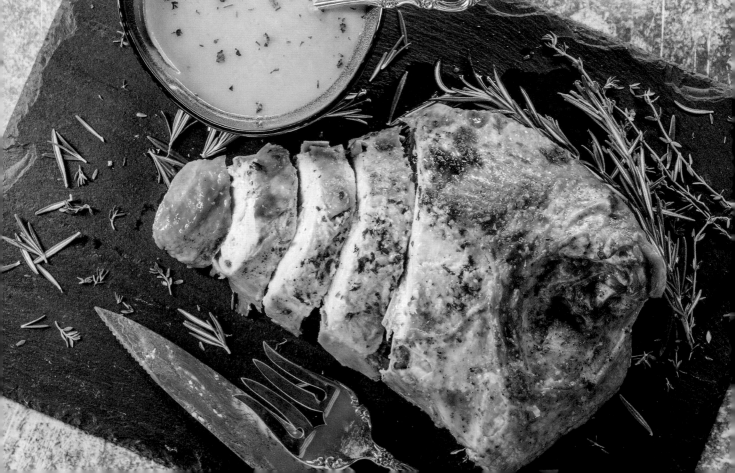

PREP TIME: **10 MINUTES** • COOKING TIME: **50 MINUTES** • MAKES: **3 SERVINGS**

BUTTER-BASTED TURKEY BREAST
WITH GRAVY

Not everyone has a big crazy family that gets together on Thanksgiving, but you still need to get your turkey on. Making a bone-in turkey breast is the way to go! It's much easier than trying to cook a fifteen-pound bird and takes less than an hour. The secret to juicy, flavorful breast meat is butter—lots and lots of butter.

 Tip | I highly recommend buying a Polder digital probe thermometer on Amazon. You can find the link at www.flavcity.com/shop.

 | To watch the video tutorial for this recipe, search "FlavCity turkey breast" on YouTube.

FOR THE TURKEY BREAST:
- 1 turkey breast, bone-in and skin on
- ½ stick citrus herb butter, see page 175 for recipe.

FOR THE GRAVY:
- 3 tablespoons unsalted grass-fed butter
- ½ cup yellow onions, chopped
- 1 teaspoon fresh thyme, chopped
- 2 cloves garlic, chopped
- 1 cup chicken stock
- ½ cup heavy cream
- ¼ teaspoon xanthan gum
- ½ teaspoon fresh lemon juice
- Kosher salt and fresh pepper

Make the turkey breast. Allow the turkey breast to sit at room temperature for 1 hour before cooking. A cold breast in a hot oven will cook unevenly and be tough. Preheat oven to 350°F and make the herb butter on page 175. Use your fingers to peel the skin off the meat to make room for the butter. You may need to make a small cut with a knife first. Stuff the butter under the skin and distribute evenly. If you have room, you can add more butter and rub it all over the turkey breast. Cover a sheet tray with tin foil and season the turkey breast with a generous amount of salt on both sides and a few cracks of pepper. Add a bit more salt than you think you need—trust me here.

Place a digital probe thermometer in the deepest part of the turkey breast, making sure not to hit the bone, and roast in the oven until the internal temperature reaches 154°F, should be about 45–50 minutes. Next, turn the broiler to medium and broil until the turkey skin is golden and crispy, about 3 minutes. Don't walk away! Watch the turkey to make sure it does not burn. Remove turkey breast from the oven and allow to rest with the thermometer in for 20 minutes under loose tin foil.

Make the gravy by preheating a medium-sized pot over medium heat along with 3 tablespoons of butter. Add the onions, thyme, ¼ teaspoon salt, and a couple cracks of pepper, and cook for 7 minutes. Add the garlic and cook for 3 minutes. Add the chicken stock, heavy cream, ¼ teaspoon salt, and a couple cracks of pepper. Bring to a bare simmer and let cook for 10 minutes. Add the xanthan gum and cook until gravy reduces and begins to thicken up, adding a touch more xanthan gum if needed. Turn the heat off and add the lemon juice and check for seasoning as you may need more salt. If you want the gravy to be silky, pass it through a strainer to catch the solids.

Slice the turkey breast and serve with gravy and enjoy!

STORAGE: Both the turkey and gravy will keep in the fridge for five days or can be frozen for two to three months.

MACROS | **per 4-ounce serving of turkey:**
273 calories
0 net and total carbs
24 grams of fat
34 grams of protein
0 fiber

MACROS | **for all the gravy:**
780 calories
7.3 grams of net and total carbs
80 grams of fat
2.5 grams of protein
0 fiber

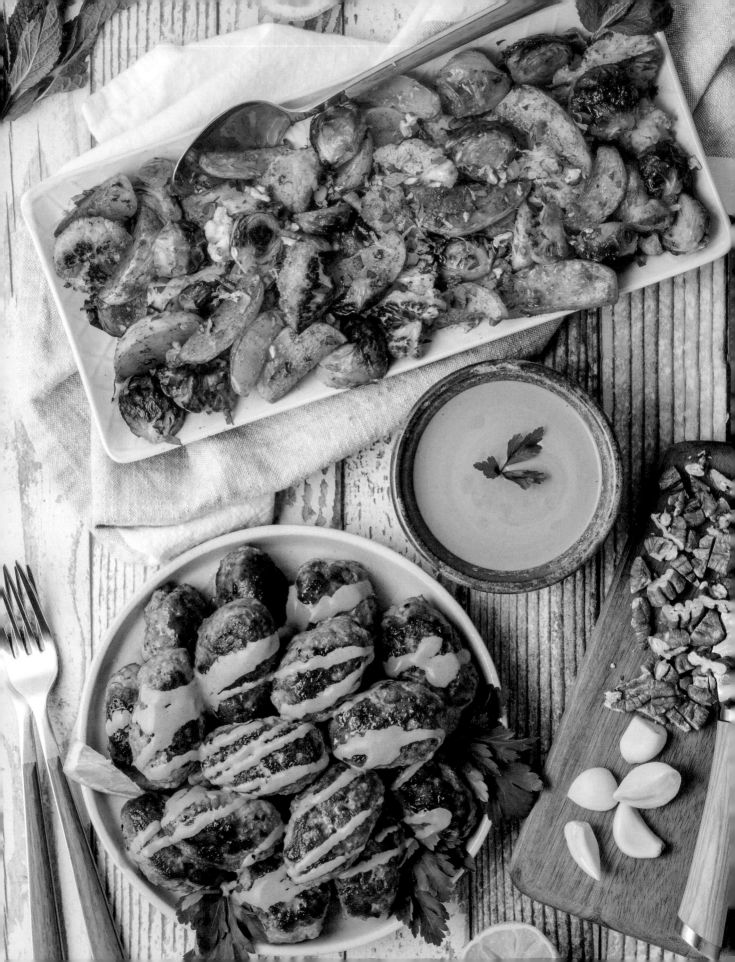

PREP TIME: **25 MINUTES** • COOKING TIME: **35 MINUTES** • MAKES: **5 MEALS**

PALEO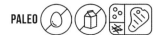

GOLDEN-SPICED TURKEY KEFTA
AND FUNKY ROASTED VEGGIES

If your taste buds have been hibernating due to a lack of flavor in your cooking, this is the recipe you need to wake them up. The number of fresh herbs and spices in this meal prep will make you feel like you are travelling down the silk road of deliciousness. Juicy turkey kefta with a drizzle of golden turmeric sauce, served with roasted and spiced veggies that are popping with flavor and texture.

FOR THE GOLDEN TAHINI SAUCE:

- ¼ cup tahini
- 1–1½ teaspoons turmeric powder
- Zest and juice of ½ lemon
- 2 drops liquid stevia
- ⅓ teaspoon kosher salt
- Couple cracks of black pepper
- 3–4 tablespoons water

To watch the video tutorial for this recipe, search "FlavCity kefta" on YouTube.

FOR THE ROASTED VEGGIES:

- ¾ teaspoon ground cumin
- ¾ teaspoon smoked paprika
- ½ teaspoon ground coriander
- ¼ teaspoon cayenne pepper
- ¼ teaspoon ground cinnamon
- 1 medium-sized head of cauliflower, cut into bite-size florets
- 1½ pounds turnips, peeled and sliced in quarters lengthwise
- 10 ounces brussels sprouts, halved
- 2 tablespoons chopped pecans
- 1 tablespoon fresh mint, chopped
- 1 tablespoon parsley, chopped
- Zest of 1 lemon
- Kosher salt
- Olive or avocado oil

FOR THE KEFTA:

- 2 pounds ground turkey thighs
- 2 cloves garlic, finely grated or chopped
- 1 tablespoon parsley, chopped
- 1 tablespoon fresh mint, chopped
- ¼ cup finely diced red onions
- 1½ teaspoons ground cumin
- 1½ teaspoons smoked paprika
- 1 teaspoon ground coriander
- ½ teaspoon cayenne pepper
- Heaping ¼ teaspoon ground cinnamon
- ¼ cup chopped pecans
- Kosher salt
- Olive or avocado oil

For the roasted veggies, preheat oven to 450°F. In a small bowl, combine the cumin, paprika, coriander, cayenne, cinnamon, and mix well. Place the cauliflower, turnips, and brussels sprouts on a sheet tray and coat with 2 tablespoons of olive oil, the spice rub, and 1 teaspoon of salt. Toss well using your hands and cook in the oven for 30 minutes or until the cauliflower is well charred on the tips. Remove from oven and add the pecans, parsley, mint, and lemon zest. Mix well and set aside.

For the kefta, add the ground turkey to a large mixing bowl along with 1½ teaspoons of salt and the remaining ingredients except the oil. Mix until just combined. Wet your hands slightly and form the mixture into small kefta that are about two inches long and one inch wide. Place them on a platter or tray. Once the kefta are formed, preheat a large pan, preferably cast-iron, over medium heat for 2 minutes with 1 tablespoon of oil. Cook for 4–5 minutes on the first side. You may need a spatula to help loosen them when you are ready to flip. Cook for another 4–5 minutes on the other side. Work in batches to not overcrowd the pan; that way the kebabs will get nice and crusty. Finish cooking all kefta and set aside. If you are not sure the kefta are cooked through—cut one in half and check.

To make the golden tahini sauce, add everything but the water to a small bowl and whisk well. Keep adding water until the sauce is pourable and not so thick. Check for seasoning as you may need a little more lemon juice.

Serve the kefta with roasted veggies and golden sauce. Enjoy!

STORAGE AND REHEATING: Everything will keep in the fridge for five days or can be frozen for two to three months. Thaw and reheat in a 350°F oven for 10 minutes. You can also reheat in the microwave with a wet paper towel placed over the top of the container to help keep the food moist.

MACROS

per serving of kefta (makes 5):
354 calories
1.9 grams of net carbs
2.5 grams of total carbs
28.3 grams of fat
23.5 grams of protein
1.3 grams of fiber

MACROS

for all the turmeric sauce:
365 calories
8.4 grams of net carbs
14.71 grams of total carbs
31.6 grams of fat
10.5 grams of protein
5.6 grams of fiber

MACROS

per serving of veggies (makes 5):
178 calories
12.1 grams of net carbs
19.3 grams of total carbs
10.1 grams of fat
5.8 grams of protein
7.3 grams of fiber

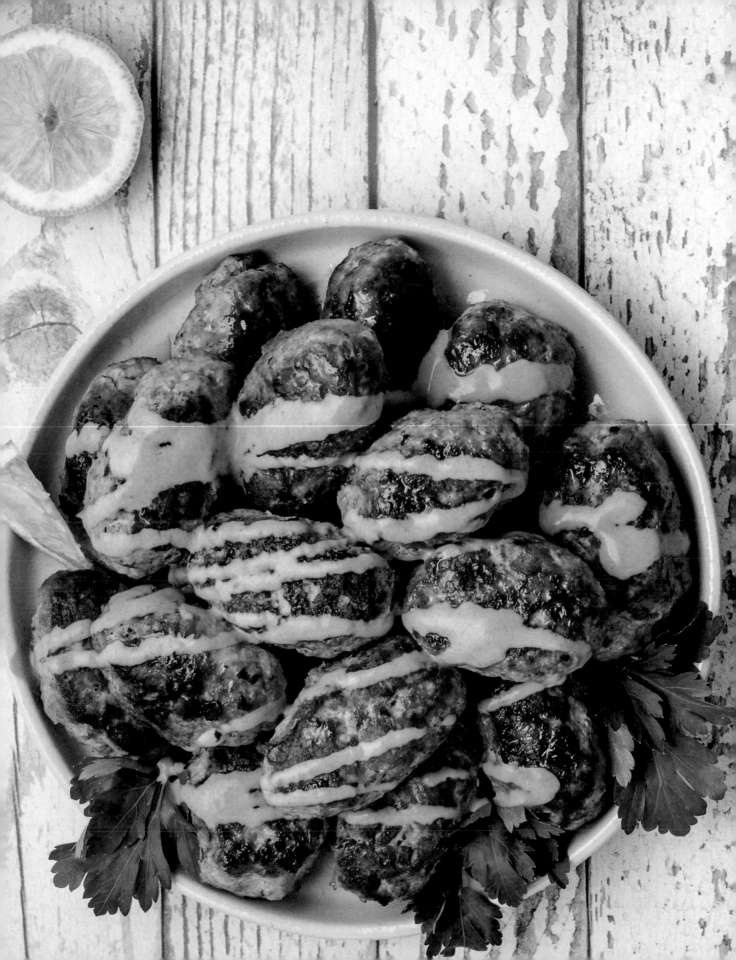

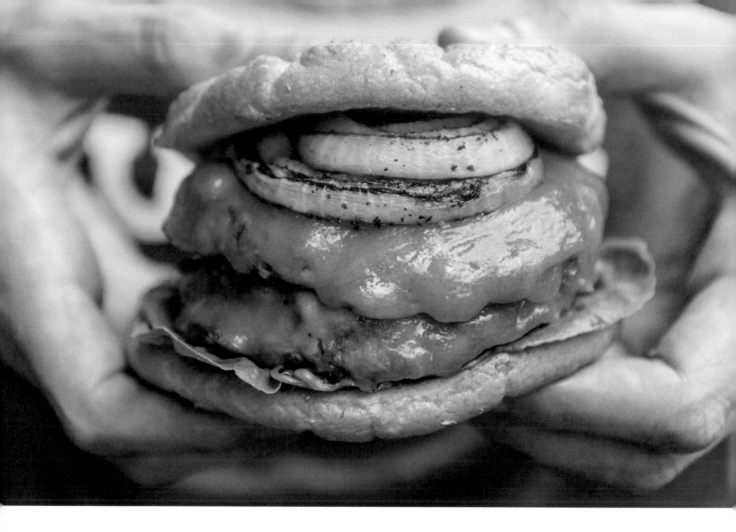

★★★★★

"Literally made this today pretty much right after watching the video. Thank you! I don't typically like ground turkey, so I loved the thigh suggestion." **—Christina Y.**

PREP TIME: **15 MINUTES** • COOKING TIME: **35 MINUTES** • MAKES: **4 BURGER PATTIES AND 4 BUNS**

DOUBLE TURKEY CHEESEBURGER
ON CLOUD BREAD BUN

You ain't gonna find this turkey burger on the menu at Shake Shack or In-N-Out Burger. This is one of a kind. Two juicy turkey patties enrobed in melted cheddar cheese, topped with spice-crusted grilled onions, and nestled between two low-carb pillowy buns. Someone, get me a chocolate shake stat!

To watch the video tutorial for this recipe, search "FlavCity turkey burger" on YouTube.

FOR THE TURKEY BURGERS:

- 1 pound ground turkey thighs
- ½ teaspoon smoked paprika
- ½ teaspoon ancho chili powder
- ½ teaspoon cumin
- 1 sweet onion
- 4 slices full-fat cheddar cheese
- Avocado oil
- Kosher salt and fresh pepper

FOR THE CLOUD BREAD:

- See recipe on page 171

For the burgers, divide the ground turkey meat into four portions. To make uniform burger patties, place a layer of plastic wrap on top of a large mayo or peanut butter lid (3.5 inches wide). Lightly pack the ground turkey into the lid and then lift the plastic wrap up so the patty comes right out. Use your hands to form a thin and uniform patty, then move it to a platter. Repeat with remaining ground turkey, making sure each patty is the same size. Place the formed burger patties in the fridge for at least 15 minutes.

Make the cloud bread buns by following the recipe on page 171.

Preheat your grill on high for 10 minutes. Combine the paprika, ancho, and cumin in a small bowl and mix well. Cut the onion into ¼ inch thick rounds, no need to peel. Drizzle 1 teaspoon of oil and rub it on both sides of the onion rounds. Season the onion rounds with a pinch of salt and a generous pinch of spice rub on each side. Grill the onions for 7–8 minutes on each side, or until slightly charred and soft. Remove and set aside.

Season the cold turkey burgers with a generous pinch of salt and a couple cracks of pepper on one side. Make sure the grill is hot, spray or brush some oil on the grill grates, and place the salted side of the burger down. Season the top side of the burger with more salt and pepper and allow to cook for 4–5 minutes. When juices start to pool on top and the edges of the burger are white, flip and immediately put the cheese slices on the burgers. Close the lid and cook another 4–5 minutes so the cheese can melt evenly. Remove from grill and let rest on a clean platter for 2 minutes. Assemble the burger with grilled onions and toppings of your choice and enjoy!

MACROS

per double burger with bun (makes 2 burgers):
739 calories
5.3 grams of net carbs
5.9 grams of total carbs
40.7 grams of fat
53 grams of protein
0.6 grams of fiber

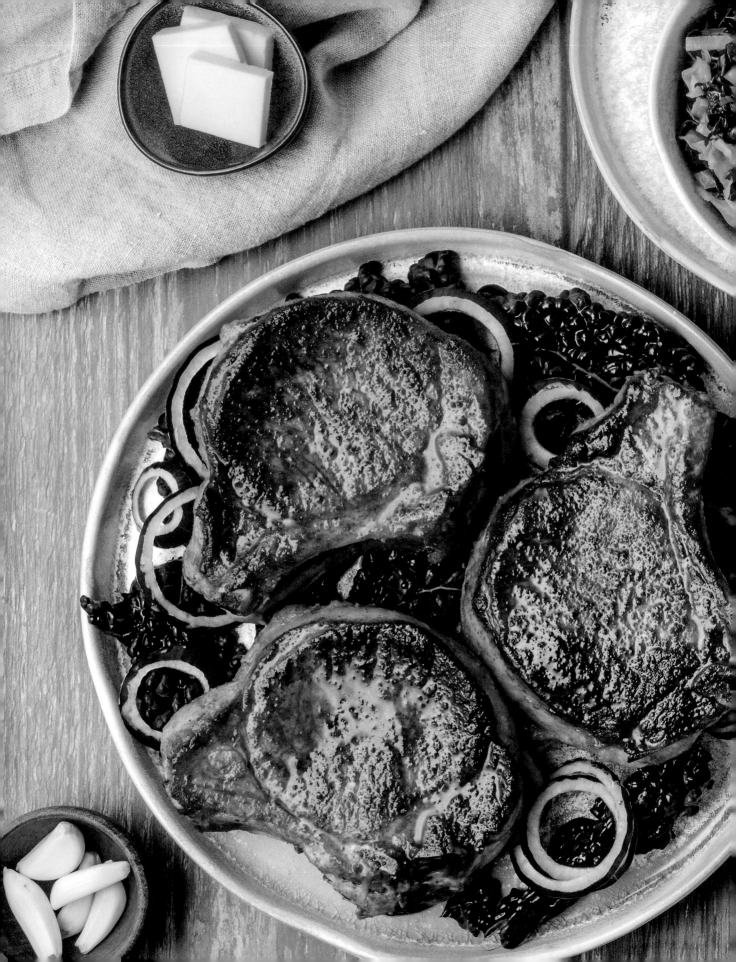

PORK—YOUR ONE STOP CHOP

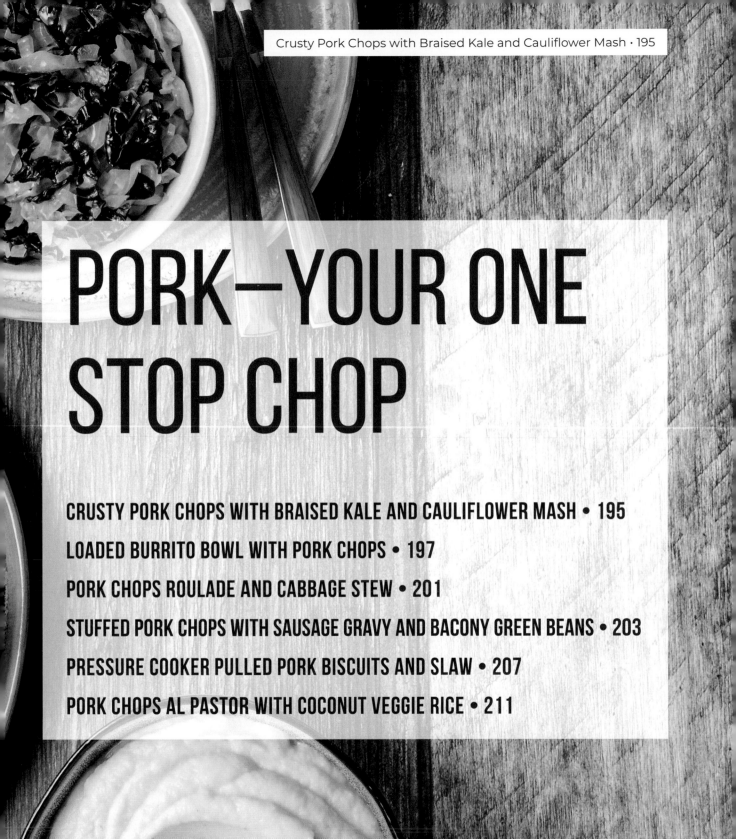

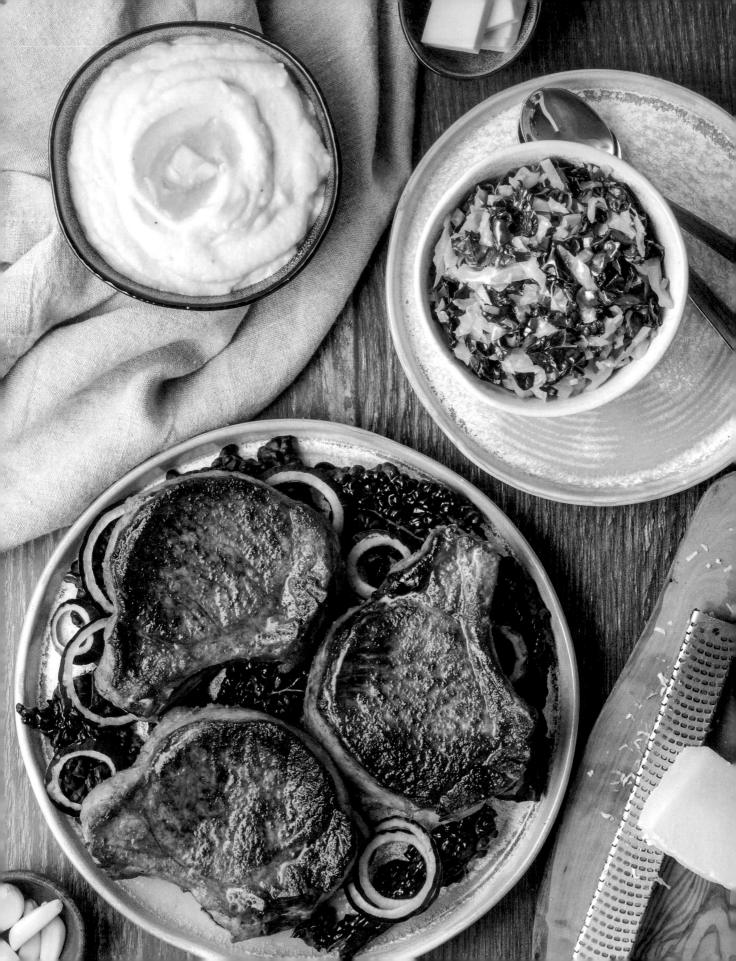

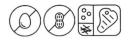

PREP TIME: **20 MINUTES** • COOKING TIME: **40 MINUTES** • MAKES: **5 MEALS**

CRUSTY PORK CHOPS
WITH BRAISED KALE AND CAULIFLOWER MASH

This here is some serious keto comfort food! Juicy spice-crusted pork chops with cheesy cauliflower mash and the most delightful spin on Southern-braised collard greens.

To watch the video tutorial for this recipe, search "FlavCity pork chops" on YouTube.

FOR THE PORK CHOPS:
- 1 teaspoon turmeric powder
- 1 teaspoon coriander
- 1 teaspoon smoked paprika
- ½ teaspoon cayenne pepper
- 5 eight-ounce, thick-cut pork chops, at least one inch thick
- Kosher salt
- Avocado oil

FOR THE BRAISED KALE:
- ½ onion, finely diced
- 3 cloves garlic, minced
- 7 ounces black (lacinato) kale, stems removed and roughly chopped
- ½ head green cabbage, finely sliced
- 1½ cups water
- 1 tablespoon plus 1 teaspoon hot sauce
- 4–6 drops of liquid stevia
- 3–4 tablespoons raw apple cider vinegar
- Kosher salt and fresh pepper
- Avocado or olive oil

FOR THE CAULIFLOWER MASH:
- See recipe on page 239

Make the spice rub for the pork chops by combining the paprika, turmeric, coriander, and cayenne pepper in a small bowl and mixing well. Season the pork chops with a generous pinch of salt and spice rub on both sides. Let sit at room temperature for 20–30 minutes.

For the braised kale, preheat a large and wide pot or Dutch oven over medium heat with 1 tablespoon of oil. Add the onions along with ¼ teaspoon of salt and a couple cracks of fresh pepper, cook for 5 minutes. Add the garlic and cook for 3 more minutes. Add the chopped kale, cabbage, ½ teaspoon salt, few cracks of pepper, and the water. Bring to a simmer and cook for 15 minutes. Add the hot sauce, stevia, vinegar, and cook another 10–15 minutes or until the veggies are soft, but still have a little bite left. Add more water if the veggies get dry. You want there to be a little bit of liquid. Check for seasoning; you want the flavors to be spicy, sweet, and tangy. Turn the heat off and set aside.

Make the cauliflower mash according to the instructions on page 239.

To cook the pork chops, preheat oven to 400°F. Preheat a large cast-iron pan over medium-high heat with 1 tablespoon of oil for 3 minutes. Sear the pork chops for 2 minutes on one side. If you don't have a large pan, do this in two batches. Flip the pork chops and immediately transfer the pan to the oven and cook for 10–12 minutes. If you have a probe thermometer, pull the chops out when the internal temperature reaches 145°F. Let the chops rest for 5 minutes so the juices can redistribute.

Plate pork chops with some of the braised kale-cabbage and the cauliflower mash and enjoy!

STORAGE: Everything will last in the fridge for five days or can be frozen for two to three months. When time to reheat, thaw and place in a 350°F oven for 10 minutes. If using the microwave, cover the container with a wet paper towel so the pork does not dry out.

MACROS

per pork chop:

328 calories
0.8 grams of net carbs
1.2 grams of total carbs
20.8 grams of fat
33 grams of protein
0 fiber

MACROS

per serving of mash (makes 5):

91 calories
4.5 grams of net carbs
8 grams of net carbs
4.4 grams of fat
5.2 grams of protein
4.2 grams of fiber

MACROS

per serving of kale and cabbage (makes 5):

66 calories
6.8 grams of net carbs
9.3 grams of total carbs
3.2 grams of fat
3.1 grams of protein
2.4 grams of fiber

★★★★★

"I finally made the cauliflower mash, and OMG this is amazing. I didn't have Parmesan cheese, so I used asiago and wow! We are loving your channel! Thank you for these recipes. Easy-peasy and delicious for this mommy of three." —**Grace R.**

"Made the pork chops and they were great! Yum!" —**Diana C.**

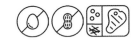

PREP TIME: **20 MINUTES** • COOKING TIME: **30 MINUTES** • MAKES: **5 MEALS**

LOADED BURRITO BOWL
WITH PORK CHOPS

This is my low-carb take on a Chipotle burrito bowl. Mexican-style cauliflower rice topped with juicy spice-crusted pork chops and all the fixings.

FOR THE PORK CHOPS:

- 1 teaspoon ancho chili powder
- 1 teaspoon cumin
- 1 teaspoon smoked paprika
- 5 boneless pork chops, about 5 ounces each
- Avocado oil
- Kosher salt

FOR THE CAULIFLOWER RICE:

- 5 cups cauliflower rice, about 1 large head
- ½ onion, chopped
- ¼ teaspoon red pepper flakes
- 2 cloves garlic, minced
- 1 teaspoon ancho chili powder
- 1 teaspoon cumin
- 1 teaspoon smoked paprika
- ¼ cup water or chicken stock
- 1–2 tablespoons fresh cilantro or parsley, chopped
- Zest and juice of ½ lime
- Avocado oil
- Kosher salt and fresh pepper

FOR THE TOPPINGS:

- 1–2 avocados
- 1 red or green bell pepper (not peppers), diced
- 5 cups of romaine lettuce, finely sliced
- 2 medium-sized tomatoes, diced
- ½ cup full-fat sour cream
- ½ cup full-fat shredded cheese, like jack or mozzarella

Tip | Avoid buying pre-grated cauliflower rice; it's full of dry stalks and the texture is much better if you do it yourself on the largest setting of a box grater.

You Tube | To watch the video tutorial for this recipe, search "FlavCity burrito bowl" on YouTube.

Make the spice rub for the pork chops by combining the paprika, ancho, and cumin in a small bowl and mix well. Season the pork chops with a generous pinch of salt and spice rub on both sides, making sure to rub the spices all around and then drizzle on 1 tablespoon oil. Let the pork chops sit at room temperature for 20–30 minutes.

Start the cauliflower rice by grating the cauliflower using the largest setting on a box grater. Try to only grate the florets, not too much of the stalks. Preheat the largest pan you have just above medium heat for 2 minutes along with 1 tablespoon of oil. Add the onion, pepper flakes, ¼ teaspoon salt, and a couple cracks of pepper, and mix well. Cook for 5 minutes then add the garlic and cook 2 more minutes. Add the paprika, ancho, and cumin, and cook for 1 minute, stirring often. Add the water or chicken stock, mix well, and cook for 30 seconds. Add all the cauliflower rice, ½ teaspoon salt, and couple cracks of pepper, and mix very well. Cover the pan with a lid or a large sheet tray, and cook for 4 minutes, stirring once. Remove cover from pan and taste the rice. If the texture is too raw, cook another minute. If it feels good, turn the heat off. Add the lime zest, lime juice, cilantro/parsley, mix well, check for seasoning, and set aside.

Cook the pork chops by preheating a large pan, preferably cast-iron, over medium-high heat for 2 minutes. Add 1 tablespoon of oil, wait 20 seconds, then add half of the chops. Cook for 4–5 minutes or until a nice crust has formed, flip and cook another 4 minutes, and then remove from pan. Repeat with remaining chops. Pork chops overcook very easily, so make sure to pull them from the pan as soon as they are done.

Chop and prep the toppings ahead of time and assemble the burrito bowl the day you want to eat it or right before eating it. I like to season the chopped tomatoes with really good extra virgin olive oil, salt, and lime juice. Top the cauliflower rice with sliced pork chops and the toppings and enjoy!

STORAGE AND REHEATING: Everything will keep in the fridge for five days. The pork can be frozen for two to three months, but not the rice. The best way to reheat the rice and chops is in a 350°F oven for 8–10 minutes. If using a microwave, cover the container with a wet paper towel and make sure not to overheat or the pork will dry out.

MACROS

per serving of cauliflower rice (makes 5):
62 calories
3.7 grams of net carbs
6.5 grams of total carbs
3 grams of fat
1.6 grams of protein
3.4 grams of fiber

MACROS

per pork chop:
269 calories
0 carbs
11.1 grams of fat
36.8 grams of protein
0 fiber

MACROS

per serving of all toppings (makes 5):
241 calories
4.94 grams of net carbs
11 grams of total carbs
20.8 grams of fat
6.2 grams of protein
5.65 grams of fiber

★★★★★

"Loved this recipe!!! It felt like I was eating a traditional burrito bowl but without the carbs! The tip to add lime juice, salt, and olive oil on the tomatoes is brilliant!! So happy I discovered this, I'll going to make it regularly." —**Natalie**

"Finally decided to try cauliflower, and I must say…this turned out amazing!!! Great flavors all around and extremely delicious! I was really surprised at how tasty the cauliflower rice was and that I ate the entire serving. Also, your videos make it very easy and enjoyable to follow along. I'll definitely make this again and look forward to making another dish from your website. Thank you so much!" —**Sal**

"I make this weekly now! I never have enough to meal prep with because I share with so many friends! LOVE LOVE LOVE!" —**Casey L.**

"For someone that does not like cauliflower, I was amazed at how delicious this actually was. It is all about adding a variety of flavors to our veggies! I definitely plan on preparing this meal in the future. It was absolutely delish!" —**Miriam**

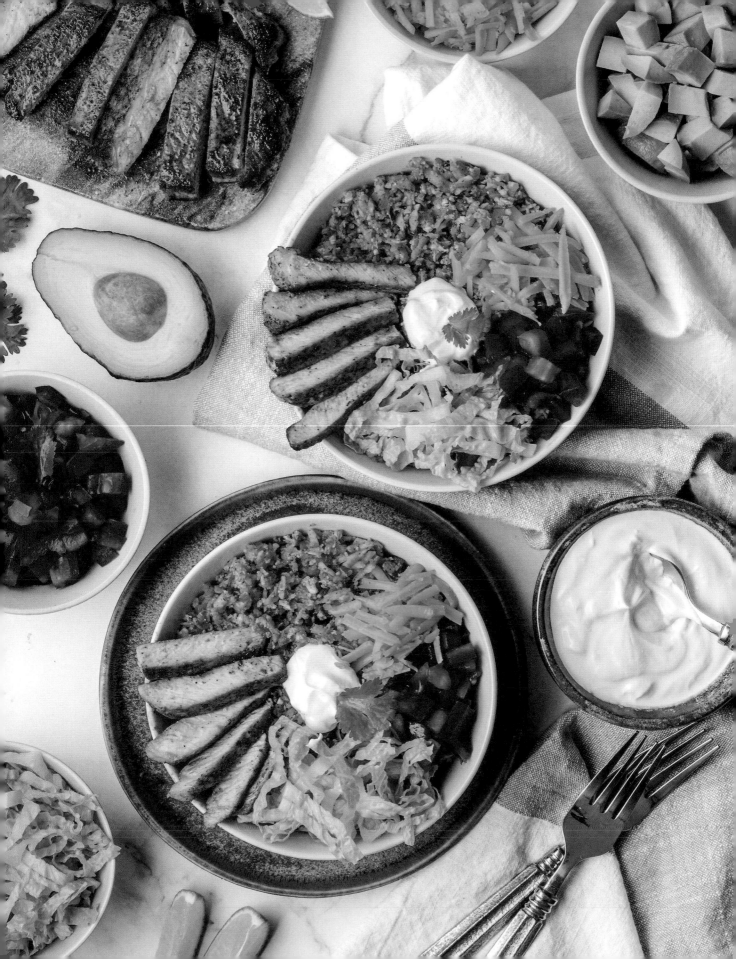

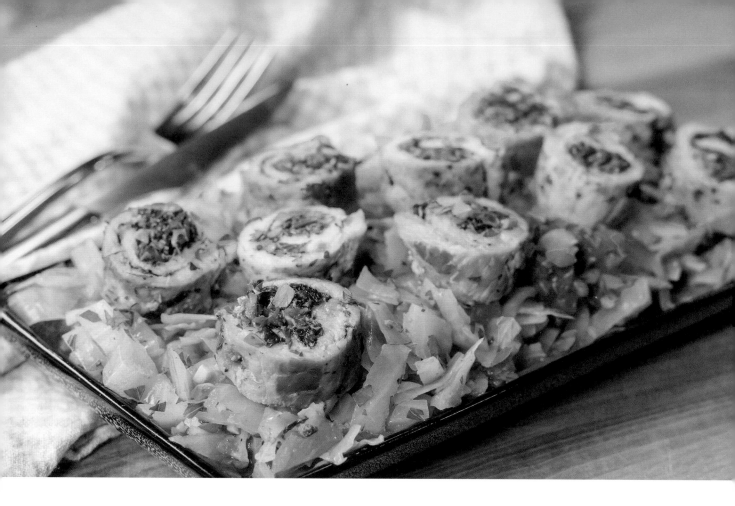

PREP TIME: **15 MINUTES** • COOKING TIME: **70 MINUTES** • MAKES: **5 SERVINGS**

PALEO / WHOLE30

PORK CHOPS ROULADE
AND CABBAGE STEW

Dessi loves a good cabbage stew cooked in a big Dutch oven. We call this type of recipe a mangia. **This one is loaded with tender cabbage cooked in tomatoes and juicy rolled pork chops stuffed with spinach and olives. It's a big pot of goodness that's going to make the house smell great.**

Tip

Make sure to buy thin-cut pork chops and pound them thinner so you can stuff and roll them. You can ask the butcher at the grocery store to do this for you.

You Tube

To watch the video tutorial for this recipe, search "FlavCity stuffed pork chops and cabbage" on YouTube.

FOR THE CABBAGE:

- 1 yellow onion, chopped
- ¼ teaspoon red pepper flakes
- 1 head of green cabbage, about 3½ pounds
- 3 cloves garlic, minced
- 1½ teaspoons sweet paprika
- 14-ounce can of San Marzano tomatoes, chopped with juice
- 3–4 cups chicken stock/broth
- 2 tablespoons chopped parsley
- 2 tablespoons chopped dill
- Olive oil
- Kosher salt and fresh pepper

FOR THE PORK:

- 10 thin-cut pork chops, about 2 pounds
- 3 ounces baby spinach
- 3 tablespoons chopped pecans
- ½ cup pitted Kalamata olives
- Zest of one lemon
- 1 tablespoon chopped parsley
- 1 tablespoon chopped dill
- Olive oil
- Kosher salt and fresh pepper

For the cabbage, preheat a large and wide pot over medium heat with 2 teaspoons of oil. Add the chopped onions, red pepper flakes, ½ teaspoon salt, and a few cracks of pepper, and cook for 10 minutes. Meanwhile, carefully cut the cabbage in half and then in half again. Slice it thin so you have shredded cabbage. Add the minced garlic and paprika to the pot and cook for 3 minutes. Add the chopped tomatoes, sliced cabbage, 1 teaspoon of salt, and a few cracks of pepper, and mix well. Add enough chicken stock to come halfway up the level of the cabbage and mix well. Bring to a boil, then reduce to a simmer and place a lid on the pot. Cook for 45–60 minutes or until the cabbage is soft. Check for seasoning after 30 minutes as you will need more salt. Add more liquid if you need it.

Make the pork roulade. Pound the pork chops very thin or ask the butcher to do this for you so you can stuff and roll them. Set aside. Make the filling for the pork by adding the spinach, pecans, olives, zest, dill, parsley, ¼ teaspoon salt, and a few cracks of pepper on a large cutting board. Use a knife to chop everything together until the spinach is wilted down and the ingredients are well combined. Season the pork chops with a pinch of salt and a couple cracks of pepper on both sides. Add some filling to each of the pork chops and tightly roll them up. Secure the rolled chops with two toothpicks. It's best to place most of the filling toward the front of the pork chops and then begin rolling.

Preheat a large non-stick pan just below high heat along with 1 tablespoon of oil. Make sure the pan is hot and add the rolled pork chops. Cook for 1–2 minutes or until deep golden brown in color. Flip and repeat and remove pork chops from pan. After the cabbage has been cooking for 1 hour and is soft, add the pork chops to the pot, nestle them down into the liquid, and cook for 10 minutes with the lid on the pot. Remove from heat and add the chopped parsley and dill.

Serve the pork chops with the cabbage and enjoy!

STORAGE: Everything will keep in the fridge for five days or can be frozen for two to three months. The best way reheat is to first thaw the meal and then place it in a 350°F oven for 7–10 minutes. If using the microwave, cover the container with a wet paper towel and make sure not to heat to high otherwise the pork will dry out.

MACROS

per serving of pork chops (makes 5):
370 calories
1.1 grams of net carbs
2.5 grams of total carbs
18.2 grams of fat
40.2 grams of protein
1.9 grams of fiber

MACROS

per serving of cabbage (makes 5):
106 calories
10.8 grams of net carbs
17.1 grams of total carbs
3.6 grams of fat
4.8 grams of protein
6 grams of fiber

PREP TIME: **25 MINUTES** • COOKING TIME: **30 MINUTES** • MAKES: **5 MEALS**

STUFFED PORK CHOPS WITH SAUSAGE GRAVY
AND BACONY GREEN BEANS

This is good old Southern comfort food done keto. The pork chops are stuffed with ricotta cheese, fried, and baked in the oven then smothered with sausage gravy and served with blistered green beans and bacon.

Tip Buy bone-in or boneless pork chops that are thick enough to stuff—at least one inch thick and about a half pound each. You can ask the butcher at the meat counter to cut a pocket for the ricotta filling if you don't feel comfortable doing that yourself.

You Tube To watch the video tutorial for this recipe, search "FlavCity stuffed pork chops" on YouTube.

FOR THE PORK CHOPS:
- ½ cup plus 2 tablespoons whole milk ricotta cheese
- 1–2 teaspoons fresh chopped parsley
- Zest of ½ lemon
- 5 thick-cut pork chops, bone-in optional
- 1 cup almond flour
- 1 teaspoon onion powder
- 1 teaspoon garlic powder
- 2 eggs
- Kosher salt and fresh pepper
- Avocado oil

FOR THE SAUSAGE GRAVY:
- 6 ounces spicy Italian sausage
- ¾ cup heavy cream
- 3 ounces cream cheese
- Kosher salt and fresh pepper
- Avocado oil

FOR THE GREEN BEANS:
- ¼ pound thick-cut bacon
- 1 pound green beans or haricot verts
- 2 tablespoons pecans, chopped
- Zest and juice of ½ lemon
- Kosher salt and fresh pepper

For the pork chops, preheat oven to 400°F, place the ricotta cheese in a medium-sized bowl, add the lemon zest, parsley, ¼ teaspoon of salt, and a couple cracks of pepper, and mix well. Use a knife to cut a pocket in the pork chops for the stuffing. Add 2 tablespoons of filling and make sure it's evenly distributed in the pork chops. Repeat this process with the remaining chops. Add the almond flour to a dish big enough to fit one pork chop, season the flour with garlic and onion powder, ½ teaspoon salt, and a few cracks of pepper, and mix well. Place the eggs in another dish along with 1 tablespoon of water and whisk well. Season both sides of the pork chops with a generous pinch of salt and a few cracks of pepper. One at a time, dredge the chops in the eggs, making sure to thoroughly coat and shake off any excess. Then place the chop in the almond flour mixture, make sure it is well coated on all sides, and move it to a sheet tray with a wire rack (if you have one). Repeat with remaining chops. Allow the chops to sit at room temperature for 20 minutes so the almond flour can really stick to the chops—this will make the crust crispy. Meanwhile, add enough oil to a pan to come halfway up the side of the chops and preheat.

Make the sausage gravy by preheating a medium-sized pan over medium-high heat. Add 1 teaspoon of oil. When the pan is hot, add the sausage, making sure to break it up into small pieces. Cook for 5 minutes until the sausage is well browned and then add the cream and a couple cracks of black pepper. Bring to a simmer and cook for 5 minutes, then add the cream cheese and cook until the mixture has thickened to a gravy consistency. You can add more cream cheese if needed. Remove from heat and set aside. Check for seasoning—you may need a pinch of salt.

Start the green beans by cutting the bacon into large cubes and placing them in a large pan, preferably cast-iron. Cook over medium heat until the bacon has rendered most its fat and has become crispy, turning down the heat if needed. Remove bacon from pan, leave fat, and turn off heat. Come back to the green beans later and proceed with the pork chops.

Once the oil has come to 350°F, **it's time to fry the chops**. You can drop a little almond flour in the oil, and it should sizzle. If not, raise the temperature a bit. Add two or three pork chops to the pan. If the oil does not sizzle, then it's not hot enough. Cook for 3–5 minutes or until golden, then flip and repeat. Place pork chops back on the rack in the sheet tray, and fry remaining chops. Transfer the chops to the oven and cook for 12–14 minutes or until the internal temperature is 150°F. Remove chops from oven and allow to rest 5–10 minutes before eating.

While the chops are frying/roasting, **make the green beans** by preheating the cast-iron pan with the bacon fat over medium-high heat for 2 minutes. Add a little more oil to the pan if there is not enough bacon fat and then add the green beans. Cook for 5–8 minutes or until blistered on the outside, but still a bit crunchy in the middle. Turn the heat off and add the pecans, lemon zest and juice, cooked bacon, ¼ teaspoon salt, and a couple cracks of pepper, and mix well. Remove green beans from the hot pan or they will overcook.

Serve the chops with the sausage gravy poured over the top and some green beans of the side.

STORAGE AND REHEATING: Everything will keep in the fridge for five days but can't be frozen because of the ricotta cheese and heavy cream. Reheat in a 350°F oven for 7–10 minutes along with the green beans. If using a microwave, cover the container with a wet paper towel and make sure not to overheat the pork.

MACROS

per pork chop (makes 5):
532 calories
3.2 net grams of carbs
5 grams of carbs
41.3 grams of fat
42.7 grams of protein
1.8 grams of fiber

MACROS

per servings of gravy (makes 5):
276 calories
1.45 grams of net and total carbs
26.8 grams of fat
6.8 grams of protein
0 fiber

MACROS

per servings of green beans (makes 5):
170 calories
3.5 grams of net carbs
6.8 grams of total carbs
14.1 grams of fat
4.7 grams of protein
3.6 grams of fiber

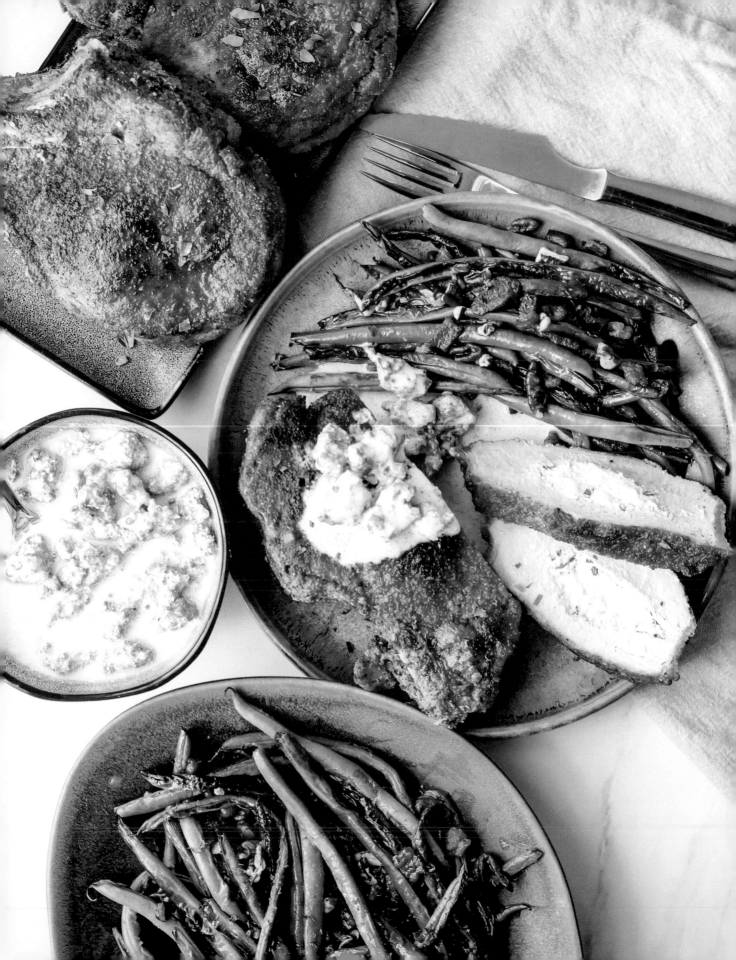

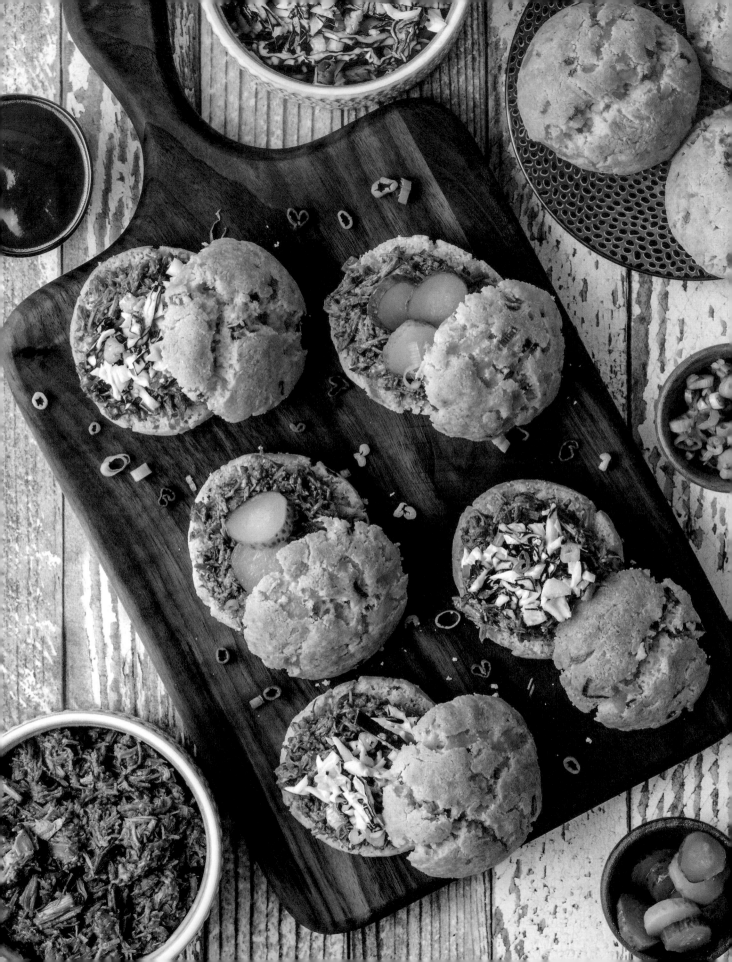

PREP TIME: **30 MINUTES** • COOKING TIME: **60 MINUTES** • MAKES: **5 MEALS**

PRESSURE COOKER
PULLED PORK BISCUITS
AND SLAW

I'll bet you thought cheesy biscuits with tender pulled pork doused in sweet and tangy BBQ sauce were off limits on keto? Well, normally you would be right. Luckily you have me as your new friend. This recipe is a bit of work, but, trust me, it's totally worth it!

 Tip | Ask the butcher to cube the pork shoulder into two-inch cubed pieces for you. This will save loads of time and they are more than happy to do it for you.

 Tip | If you don't have an electric pressure cooker, follow the recipe and braise the pork for 2½ hours with the lid closed on the stovetop or in a 325°F oven. You can also slow cook for 8 hours.

 Tip | If you want to save time, feel free to buy your favorite bottle of keto BBQ sauce. Just make sure it has no added sugar. You can also buy a big bag of slaw mix instead of shredding the cabbage yourself.

 You Tube | To watch the video tutorial for this recipe, search "FlavCity keto pulled pork" on YouTube.

FOR THE BBQ SAUCE:
- 1 cup sugar-free ketchup
- 4½ tablespoons Sukrin brown sugar substitute or monk fruit sweetener
- ½ cup water
- 1 tablespoon tamari soy sauce
- 1 tablespoon Worcestershire sauce
- 1 tablespoon stone-ground or Dijon mustard
- 3 tablespoons apple cider vinegar
- 1 teaspoon garlic powder
- 1 teaspoon ancho chile powder
- 1 teaspoon onion powder
- ¼ teaspoon cayenne pepper
- 1 teaspoon liquid smoke

FOR THE BISCUITS:
- See recipe on page 159

FOR THE PORK:
- Coffee spice rub, see page 109
- 3 pounds pork shoulder, cut in 2-inch cubes
- 1¼ cup beef stock/broth
- 1–2 cups BBQ sauce
- ⅓ cup apple cider vinegar
- 1 teaspoon of hot sauce
- Kosher salt
- Avocado oil

FOR THE SLAW:
- ½ medium-sized head red cabbage
- ½ medium-sized head green cabbage
- ½ cup green onions, finely sliced
- ½ cup chopped pecans
- ¾ cup celery, sliced
- ¾ cup of full-fat, sugar-free mayonnaise
- ½ teaspoon toasted sesame oil
- 1 tablespoon tamari soy sauce
- Zest and juice of ½ lemon
- Kosher salt and fresh pepper

Make the BBQ sauce by adding all the ingredients to a medium-sized pot and bring to a low simmer. Cook for 45 minutes, stirring often. Check for seasoning, you may need more brown sugar substitute. To make the sauce extra smooth, blend or use a hand blender for 30 seconds. Sauce will keep in the fridge for 3 weeks and tastes even better the next day.

For the pork, make the coffee spice rub according to the recipe on page 109. Season the cubed pork shoulder with a generous pinch of salt and a generous amount of the spice rub. Rub the seasoning all around and set aside. Preheat electric pressure cooker to the high setting of sauté and add 1 tablespoon of oil. Wait for the oil to get hot and add ⅓ of the pork. Brown well on all sides for about 6 minutes and remove the pork and repeat with the remaining two batches, adding more oil if needed. Turn the pot off and add ¼ cup of the beef stock and use a wooden spoon to scrape the sticky bits from the bottom of the pot. Add the pork back to the pot along with 1 cup of BBQ sauce, the remaining beef stock, vinegar, and hot sauce. Mix everything very well, close the lid, and set the pot to pressure cook on high for 40 minutes. Once the time is up, allow the pot to sit for 10 minutes and then carefully release the pressure using the valve.

Make the cheddar biscuits according to the instructions on page 159.

Make the slaw by finely slicing both heads of cabbage and adding to a large bowl. Add the green onions, pecans, celery, ¼ teaspoon salt, and few cracks of pepper, and mix well. Make the dressing by adding the mayo to a bowl along with the sesame oil, tamari soy sauce, zest and lemon juice, ¼ teaspoon salt, and a couple cracks of pepper. Mix well and check for seasoning. The flavor should be tangy and bright, so add more lemon juice if needed. Only combine the dressing and slaw right before (or a few hours before) you want to enjoy it. The slaw is hearty and can be dressed and taken to work without getting soggy.

Once the pork is done cooking, transfer it to a large cutting board, leaving the cooking liquid in the pot. Roughly chop the pork to desired consistency and move to a large bowl. Add a splash of the cooking liquid to the pork and more BBQ sauce and mix well. Save 1 cup of the cooking liquid, making sure to discard the fat, and store the leftover pulled pork in a bowl with the liquid in the fridge. This will keep the pork very moist.

Make sandwiches by cutting the biscuits in half, adding some pork, and topping it off with slaw. Enjoy!

STORAGE AND REHEATING: Everything will keep in the fridge for five days. Only the biscuits and pork can be frozen for two to three months. Thaw and reheat the pulled pork in a hot pan and the biscuits in a 350°F oven for 5 minutes. If using microwave, cover the pork and biscuits with a wet paper towel and make sure not to overheat as the food will dry out.

MACROS

per serving of pulled pork (makes 5):
674 calories
5.6 grams of net carbs
6.3 grams of total carbs
37 grams of fat
75 grams of protein
Less than 1 gram of fiber

MACROS

per serving of slaw (makes 5):
342 calories
7.1 grams of net carbs
12 grams of total carbs
31.9 grams of fat
4.7 grams of protein
5.3 grams of fiber

MACROS

per biscuit (makes 10):
230 calories
1.8 net grams of carbs
3.6 grams of total carbs
22.4 grams of fat
6.2 grams of protein
1.8 grams of fiber

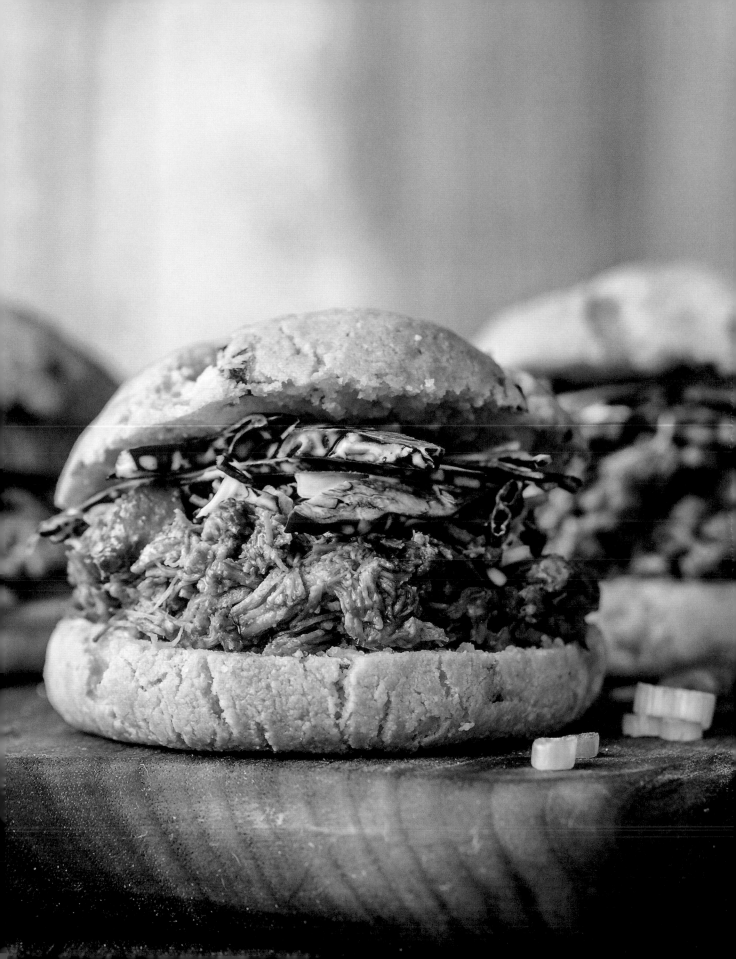

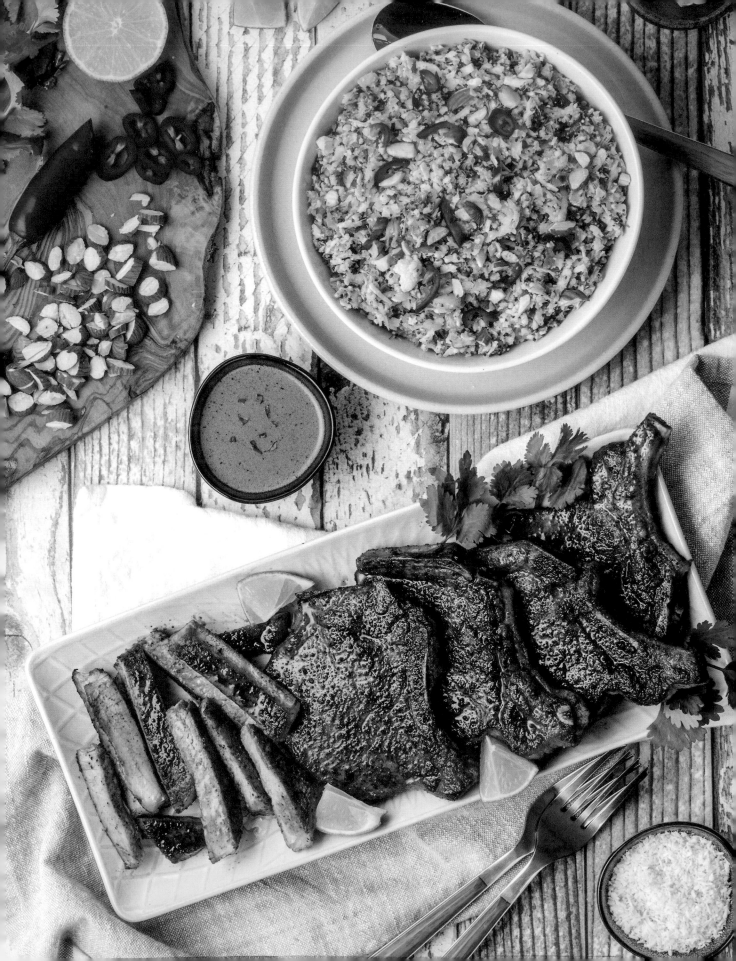

PREP TIME: **15 MINUTES** • COOKING TIME: **30 MINUTES** • MAKES: **5 MEALS**

PALEO / WHOLE30

PORK CHOPS AL PASTOR
WITH COCONUT VEGGIE RICE

Dessi and I went to Tulum and had the most epic tacos al pastor with so much meat piled on the spit—it seemed to defy logic. I was inspired from that trip to create this low-carb meal prep that has flavors and textures that are like a fiesta in your mouth. Que paso!

To watch the video tutorial for this recipe, search "FlavCity pork chops pastor" on YouTube.

FOR THE PORK CHOPS:

- 1 teaspoon ancho chili powder
- 1 teaspoon cumin
- 1 teaspoon smoked paprika
- ½ teaspoon ground coriander
- 10 thin-cut pork chops, about 2 pounds total
- 1 cup full-fat coconut milk
- Zest and juice of ½ lime
- Kosher salt
- Avocado or coconut oil

FOR THE CAULIFLOWER RICE:

- 1 large head of cauliflower
- 1½ pounds of broccoli on the stalk
- ½ a red onion, chopped
- 3 cloves garlic, minced
- 1 red finger chili, thinly sliced or a pinch of red pepper flakes
- 2 tablespoons unsweetened shredded coconut flakes
- 2 tablespoons chopped almonds or pecans, toasted if desired
- Lime zest and juice
- 2–3 tablespoons cilantro or parsley, chopped
- Kosher salt and fresh pepper
- Avocado or coconut oil

Make the spice rub for the pork chops by combining the paprika, cumin, chili powder, and coriander in a small bowl, mix well. Season the pork chops on both sides with a generous pinch of salt and spice rub. Let the pork sit at room temperature for 15–25 minutes.

Start the rice by grating the cauliflower on the large side of a box grater, making sure not to grate too much of the stalk. Next grate the broccoli, but this time grate a little of the stalk after you have grated the florets. Move the riced cauliflower and broccoli aside. Preheat a large non-stick pan over medium heat with 1 tablespoon of oil. Add the onions, garlic, chilies, ¼ teaspoon salt, and a couple cracks of pepper and cook for 7 minutes. Add the riced cauliflower, broccoli, ½ teaspoon salt, a couple cracks of pepper, and give everything a good stir. Cover the pan with a lid or a sheet tray, raise the heat just a little, and let cook for 5 minutes. Remove the lid and give the rice a taste. The raw flavor of the veggies should be gone, but you still want them to have a little crunch. Cook another minute if needed. Lower the heat to low and add the coconut flakes, nuts, zest and juice of ½ a lime, and cilantro, and mix well. Turn the heat off and check for seasoning as you may need more lime or salt. Set aside.

For the pork chops, preheat the same pan, or better yet, a large cast-iron pan, over medium-high heat for 2 minutes with 1 tablespoon of oil. Add five of the chops to the pan and cook for 3 minutes on the first side, flip, and cook another 2–3 minutes. Thin pork chops cook quickly, so make sure not to overcook them or they will get dry. Add a little more oil to the pan and cook the second batch of chops. Remove pork chops from pan and lower heat to medium. Add the coconut milk, lime zest and juice, and bring the sauce to a simmer. Let cook for 5 minutes or until reduced by almost half and pour the sauce over the cooked pork chops.

Serve the chops with leftover sauce on the side along with the rice and enjoy!

STORAGE AND REHEATING: The pork chops and riced veggies will last in the fridge for five days or you can freeze both for two to three months. Thaw and reheat in a 350°F oven for 10 minutes. If reheating in the microwave, take the lid off, cover with a wet paper towel and make sure not to reheat too long or the pork will dry out.

MACROS

per serving of pork chops (makes 5):
- 379 calories
- 1.8 grams of net carbs
- 2 grams of total carbs
- 22.3 grams of fat
- 39.4 grams of protein
- 0.2 fiber

MACROS

per serving of veggie rice (makes 5):
- 110 calories
- 5.3 grams of net carbs
- 8.1 grams of total carbs
- 8 grams of fat
- 2.8 grams of protein
- 3.3 grams of fiber

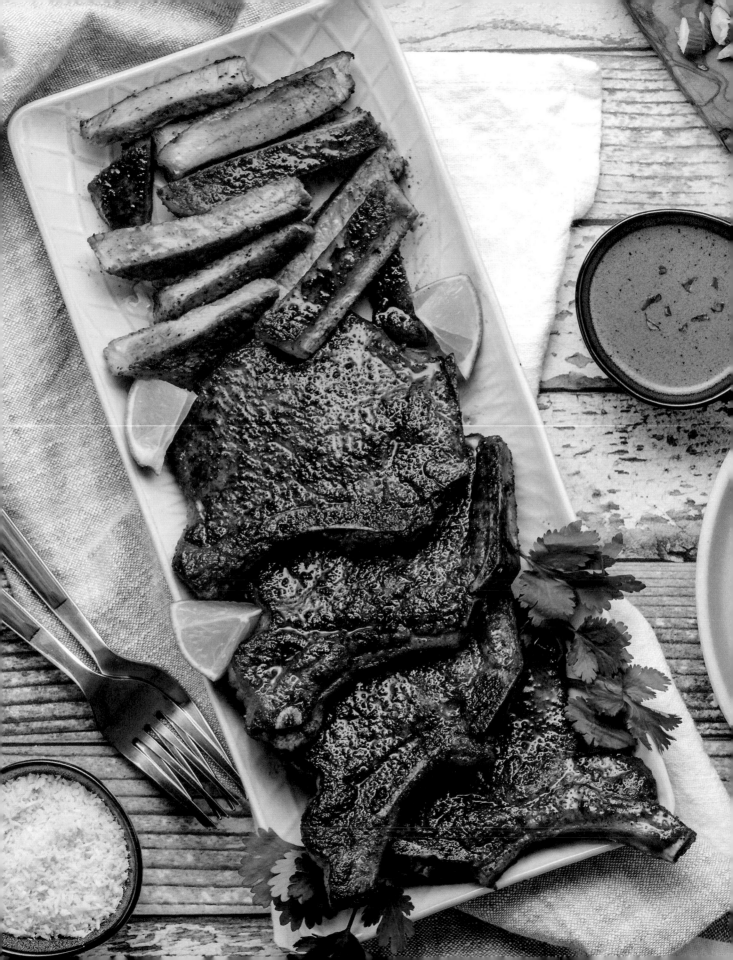

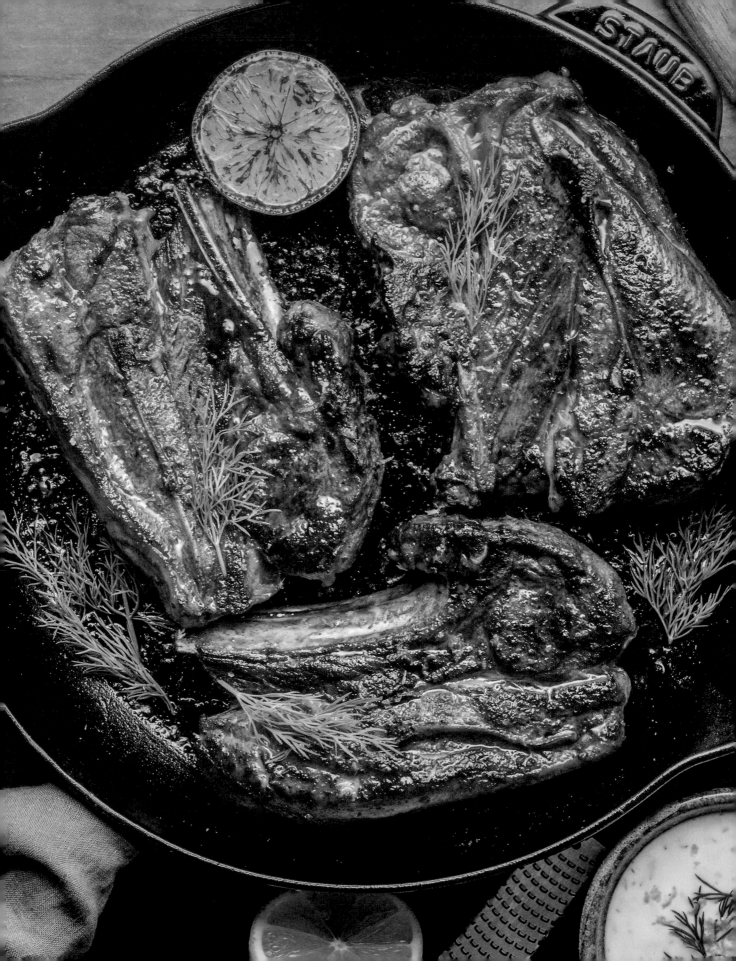

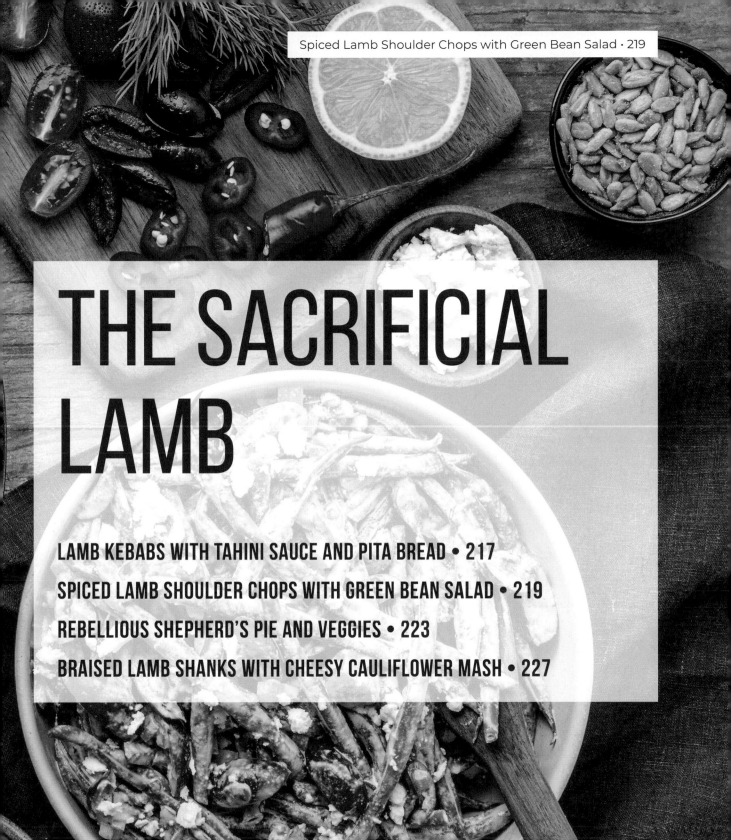

THE SACRIFICIAL LAMB

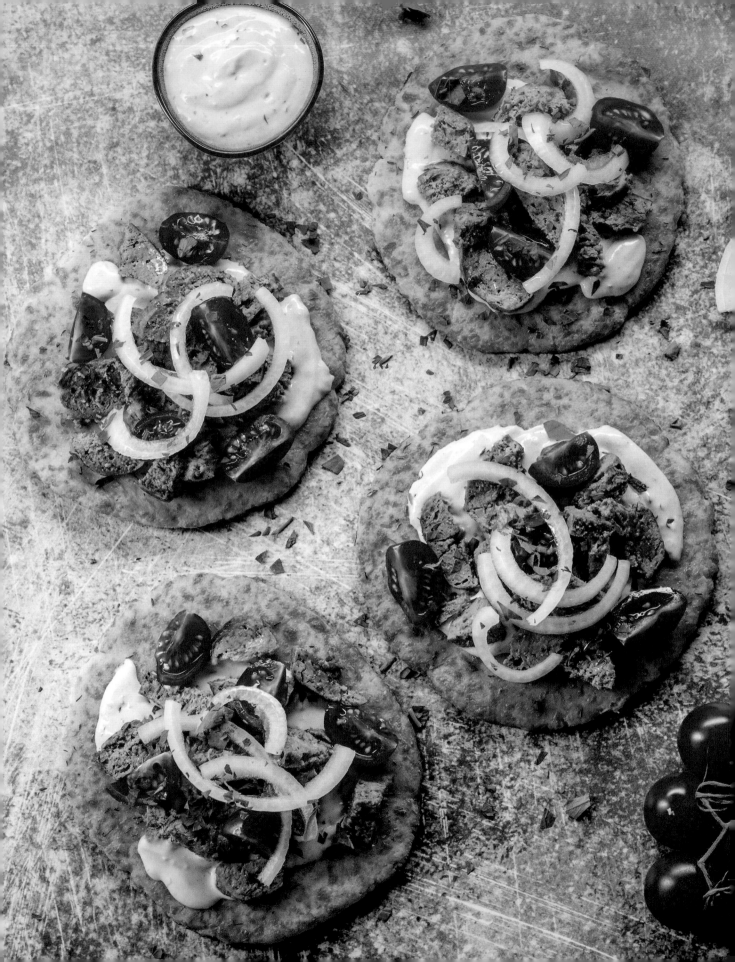

PREP TIME: **25 MINUTES** • COOKING TIME: **30 MINUTES** • MAKES: **5 MEALS**

LAMB KEBABS
WITH TAHINI SAUCE AND PITA BREAD

Dessi and I were blown away by the food on a recent trip to Jordan and Israel. The flavors were so vibrant and fresh. This is our keto take on lamb kebabs using a low-carb pita bread that is fantastic. We also learned a lot about tahini, so you may want to double the recipe and use it for roasted veggies and spreads.

To watch the video tutorial for this recipe, search "FlavCity keto kebab" on YouTube.

FOR THE KEBABS:
- 2 pounds ground lamb
- 1½ teaspoons smoked paprika
- 1½ teaspoons cumin
- 1 teaspoon ground coriander
- ½ teaspoon ground cinnamon
- ¼ teaspoon ground cloves
- ¼ teaspoon ground cardamom
- 2 cloves garlic, finely grated
- Zest of 1 lemon
- 1 tablespoon freshly chopped parsley
- 1 teaspoon dried thyme
- Kosher salt and fresh pepper
- Olive or avocado oil

FOR THE PITA BREAD:
- See recipe on page 165

FOR THE TAHINI SAUCE:
- 2 cloves garlic, finely grated
- Juice of 1 lemon
- ⅓ cup runny tahini
- ¼ teaspoon salt
- Ice water
- 1 teaspoon freshly chopped parsley

Make the kebabs by adding the ground lamb to a large bowl along with the remaining ingredients (except the oil), 1½ teaspoons salt, and a few cracks of pepper. Use your hands to mix everything well, but make sure you don't overmix as that will make the lamb tough. Form the mixture into individual kebabs about one by four inches or any size you desire, making sure they are not too fat; the recipe should make eight. Store the kebabs in the fridge for 20 minutes before cooking so they can firm up.

Make the pita bread by following instructions on page 165.

Make the tahini sauce by finely grating the garlic in a small bowl and covering with the juice of 1 lemon. Let sit for 5–15 minutes so the raw flavor of the garlic goes away. Add the tahini to a small food processor or use a handheld stick blender with a tall and narrow jar. Add the garlic and lemon juice, salt, and blend for a few seconds. Add some ice water (about 2–4 tablespoons) while blending and keep going until the texture is smooth and creamy. If you need to add more water, do so. Check for seasoning as you may need more salt. Set aside.

To cook the kebabs, preheat a large non-stick pan just below medium-high heat for 2 minutes. Add 1 tablespoon of oil, wait 10 seconds, and then add half of the kebabs and cook for 4–5 minutes. You have to work in two batches. Otherwise, you will overcrowd the pan. Once the kebabs have nice color on the first side, flip and cook another 4 minutes. To ensure the kebabs cook evenly, turn them on both of their sides and cook for 30 seconds each side. To make sure the lamb is cooked through, you can cut into one to test. Remove from pan and cook the second batch.

Serve the kebabs with the pita bread and tahini sauce and enjoy! You will have more kebabs than can fit on the pita breads, so just enjoy those with sauce.

STORAGE AND REHEATING: Everything will keep in the fridge for five days, only the kebabs and pita can be frozen for two to three months. Thaw and reheat in a 350°F oven for 7–10 minutes or covered with a wet paper towel in the microwave.

MACROS

per kebab (makes 8):
281 calories
0.7 net and total grams of carbs
26.6 grams of fat
19 grams of protein
0 fiber

MACROS

per pita bread (makes 5):
330 calories
4.35 grams of net carbs
7.95 grams of total carbs
27.2 grams of fat
16.8 grams of protein
3.6 grams of fiber

MACROS

for all the tahini sauce:
500 calories
8.8 grams of net carbs
10 grams of total grams
46 grams of fat
16.5 grams of protein
1.5 grams of fiber

★★★★★

"I absolutely loved this recipe! The lamb kebabs were a flavor bomb. I could eat those by themselves, but it would be a shame not to have them with the flatbreads." —**Adrian E.**

"Ok. This deserves a medal. It is so so delish! My store didn't have a block of mozzarella. So I got a bag of grated mozzarella and still the pita breads turned out great—very nice texture and taste. I'm making these tonight. Again!" —**Yana**

"You have by far the best keto meals on the net. I just finished my lunch, and I must say I feel so satisfied, like I just ate something from a restaurant. So delicious!!! Thank you!" —**Nina**

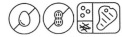

PREP TIME: **20 MINUTES** • COOKING TIME: **30 MINUTES** • MAKES: **5 MEALS**

SPICED LAMB SHOULDER CHOPS
WITH GREEN BEAN SALAD

These spice-crusted lamb shoulder chops have lots of flavor and cook up just like a steak. The chops are served with a creamy and crunchy Mediterranean green bean salad that Zeus himself would approve of.

 Tip | Lamb shoulder chops—a.k.a. blade chops—are the perfect cut for keto meal prep because they have lots of yummy fat and can be cooked just like a steak. Because they have a large bone, you may want to eat two chops per meal.

 | To watch the video tutorial for this recipe, search "FlavCity keto lamb chops" on YouTube.

FOR THE GREEN BEANS:
- 1 pound of haricot vert or green beans
- 2 tablespoons unsalted sunflower seeds
- ¼ cup pitted Kalamata olives, sliced
- 1 small red-hot chili or jalapeño pepper, thinly sliced
- ½ cup orange peppers, diced
- ½ cup cherry tomatoes, quartered lengthwise
- 3 tablespoons of tahini
- Zest and juice of ½ lemon
- 1 clove of garlic, grated
- 1 teaspoon extra virgin olive oil
- 1 teaspoon freshly chopped Italian parsley
- cold water
- Kosher salt and fresh pepper
- ¼ cup crumbled feta cheese

FOR THE LAMB:
- 1½ teaspoons smoked paprika
- 1½ teaspoons ground cumin
- ½ teaspoon dried oregano
- ½ teaspoon cayenne pepper
- ¼ teaspoon ground cinnamon
- 5–10 lamb shoulder chops
- Avocado oil
- Kosher salt

FOR THE YOGURT DIPPING SAUCE:
- ¾ cup full-fat Greek-style yogurt
- Zest and juice of ½ lemon
- 2 teaspoons freshly chopped dill
- 1 teaspoon extra virgin olive oil
- ¼ teaspoon kosher salt and a couple cracks of pepper

Make the spice rub for the lamb shoulder chops by combining the smoked paprika, cumin, oregano, cayenne, and cinnamon in a small bowl and mix well. If making ten chops, you will need to double the spice rub quantities. Season the lamb chops with a generous pinch of spice rub and salt on both sides. Let the chops sit at room temperature for 20 minutes so the marinade can infuse flavor.

Start the green bean salad by bringing a medium-sized pot of water to a boil. Add 2 teaspoons of salt to the boiling water and carefully add all the green beans or haricot vert. As soon as the beans go in the water, set a timer for 2½ minutes. While they are cooking, fill a large bowl with a bunch of ice and then add cold water. After 2½ minutes, immediately strain the beans and get them in the ice water. Move the beans around and keep them in the ice bath for 1 minute or until the beans are cold. Remove beans and allow them to drain very well before adding to a large clean bowl. Add the sunflower seeds, olives, orange peppers, sliced chili, and cherry tomatoes to the bowl with the beans and set aside.

Make the dressing by combining the tahini, lemon zest and juice, grated garlic, olive oil, and parsley. Whisk well and add just enough water, over a ¼ cup, to make the dressing pourable along with ¼ teaspoon salt and a couple cracks of pepper. Check for seasoning. You may need more lemon juice or salt. To make the salad last five days, store the dressing and bean salad separately in the fridge and only dress a single portion the day you want to eat it. Add a small pinch of salt and pepper to the bean salad, coat with just enough dressing, mix well, and add the feta cheese.

To cook the lamb shoulder chops, preheat a large cast-iron pan over medium-high heat for 2 minutes along with 1 tablespoon of oil. Once hot, add three or four chops to the pan and press down for 3 seconds so they make maximum contact with the pan. Cook for 6 minutes and flip. Turn the heat down to medium and cook 6 more minutes and remove from pan. Repeat with the next batch of chops. It is very important not to overcrowd the pan, or the chops won't get crusty, so you need to work in batches. If eating the chops immediately, allow to rest for 5 minutes so the juices can redistribute.

Make the yogurt sauce by adding all the ingredients to a small bowl and whisking well. Check for seasoning— you want the flavors to be lemony, so add more lemon juice if needed.

Serve the lamb with yogurt sauce and green bean salad. Enjoy!

STORAGE AND REHEATING: The cooked lamb shoulder chops will keep in the fridge for five days or can be frozen for two to three months. The yogurt and green beans will keep in the fridge for five days but can't be frozen. Thaw and reheat the chops in a 350°F oven for 10 minutes or covered with a wet paper towel in the microwave.

MACROS

per lamb shoulder chop:

404 calories
0 carbs
33 grams of fat
28.5 grams of protein
0 fiber

MACROS

for all the yogurt sauce:

168 calories
6.2 grams of net and total carbs
8.5 grams of fat
17.3 grams of protein
0 fiber

MACROS

per serving of green beans (makes 5):

142 calories
5.7 grams of net carbs
10.8 grams of total carbs
8.31 grams of fat
4.9 grams of protein
5.1 grams of fiber

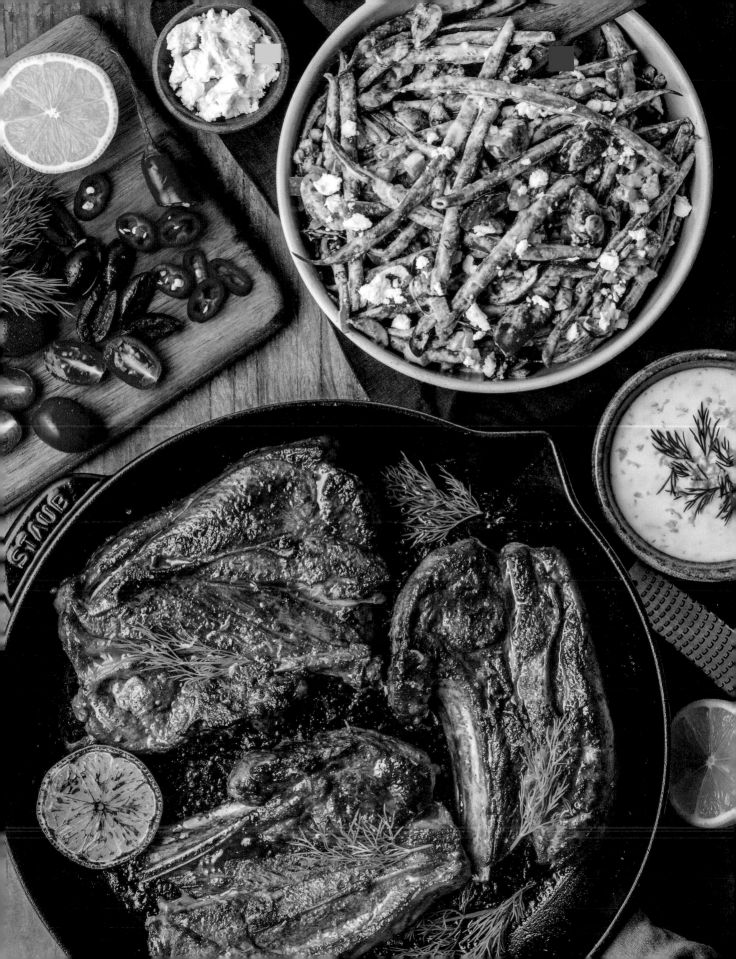

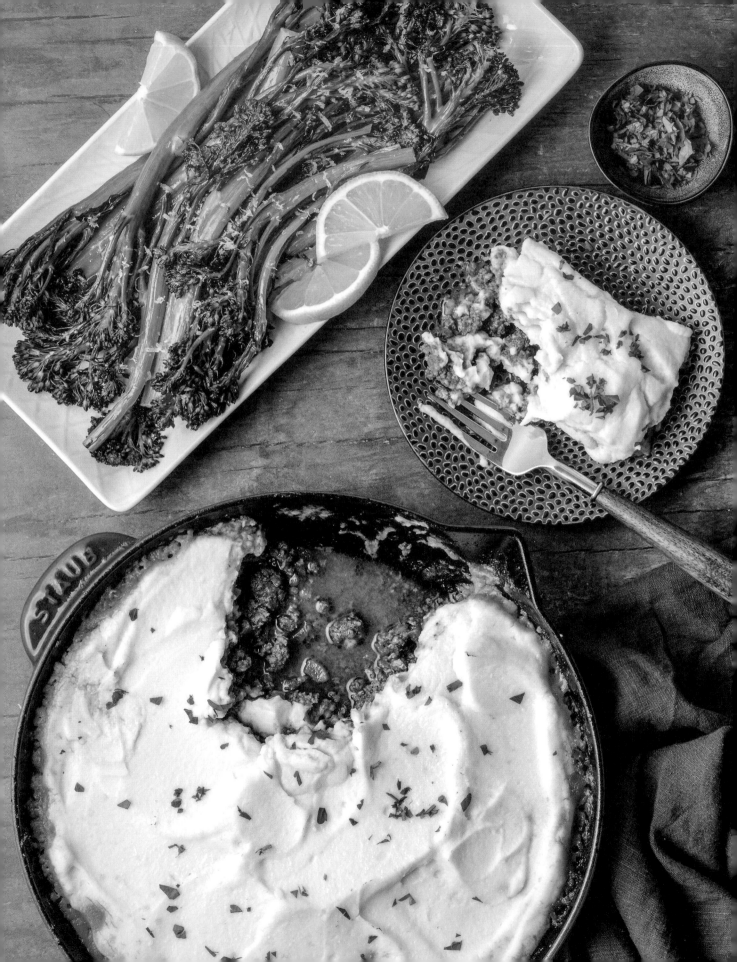

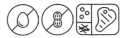

PREP TIME: **20 MINUTES** • COOKING TIME: **50 MINUTES** • MAKES: **5 MEALS**

REBELLIOUS
<u>SHEPHERD'S PIE</u>
AND VEGGIES

Comfort food alert! This meal prep is paired best with your favorite Netflix show and a comfy couch. We're serving up juicy ground lamb shepherd's pie loaded with veggies and topped with whipped cauliflower mash. Feel free to use ground beef for this recipe—then it's called a cottage pie.

Tip

The shepherd's pie should be made in a twelve- to fourteen-inch skillet or cast-iron pan, so it can go from stove top to oven. Alternatively, you can make the lamb mixture and transfer it to a nine-by-thirteen-inch baking dish.

FOR THE CAULIFLOWER MASH:

- Double the recipe for Buttery Mashed Cauliflower on page 239

FOR THE SHEPHERD'S PIE:

- ½ onion, diced
- 2 stalks celery, diced
- 1 large zucchini, diced
- 1 green bell pepper, diced
- ½ teaspoon dried thyme
- 3 cloves garlic, minced
- 2 tablespoons tomato paste
- 2 pounds ground lamb
- ¼ cup beef stock/broth
- 1 teaspoon of tamari soy sauce
- 1–2 teaspoons fresh Italian parsley, chopped
- Olive or avocado oil
- Kosher salt and fresh pepper

FOR THE BROCCOLINI:

- 1½ pounds broccolini or baby broccoli
- Zest of 1 lemon
- Olive or avocado oil
- Kosher salt and fresh pepper

Make the cauliflower mash by following the instruction on page 239. Make sure to double the recipe so there is enough topping to cover the Shepherd's pie.

To make the pie, preheat oven to 450°F and preheat a twelve- to fourteen-inch cast-iron pan or oven-safe skillet just above medium heat. Add 1 tablespoon of oil along with the onions, celery, zucchini, bell pepper, thyme, ½ teaspoon of salt, and a few cracks of pepper. Mix well and cook for 10 minutes and then add the garlic and cook until the veggies are very soft. Add the tomato paste and cook for 1 minute. Turn the heat to medium-high and add the lamb along with 1 teaspoon of salt and a few cracks of pepper. Use a spatula to break up the lamb into small pieces while it cooks. When the lamb is almost cooked through, add the beef stock and tamari and turn the heat down to low. Add 1½ teaspoons of parsley, mix well, and turn the heat off as soon as the lamb is cooked through. Press the lamb mixture evenly into the pan, pour the cauliflower mash topping over, and smooth it out to the edges. You may not need all the mash; save leftovers to eat on the side. Grate some cheese leftover from the mash over the top if desired and bake for 10 minutes. Turn the broiler to high and cook until the top is golden in spots or about 5 minutes. Remove from oven and allow to cool for 20 minutes.

Make the broccolini. As soon as the pie comes out of the oven, set the oven temperature to 450°F. Place the broccolini on a sheet tray and season with 1–2 tablespoons of oil, ½ teaspoon salt, few cracks of pepper, and mix well. Roast in the oven for 20–25 minutes or until broccolini is slightly charred on the exterior and cooked through. Remove from oven, add lemon zest right over the top, and serve with the shepherd's pie. Enjoy!

STORAGE AND REHEATING: Everything will keep in the fridge for five days or can be frozen for two to three months. Reheat in a 350°F for 10–13 minutes. If you are using a microwave, take the lid off and cover the container with a wet paper towel. This will keep the food moist.

MACROS

per serving of pie (makes 5):
697 calories
11 grams of net carbs
17.8 grams of total carbs
51 grams of fat
39.2 grams of protein
6.8 grams of fiber

MACROS

per serving of broccolini (makes 5):
94.2 calories
5.5 grams of net carbs
9 grams of total carbs
6 grams of fat
3.8 grams of protein
3.5 grams of fiber

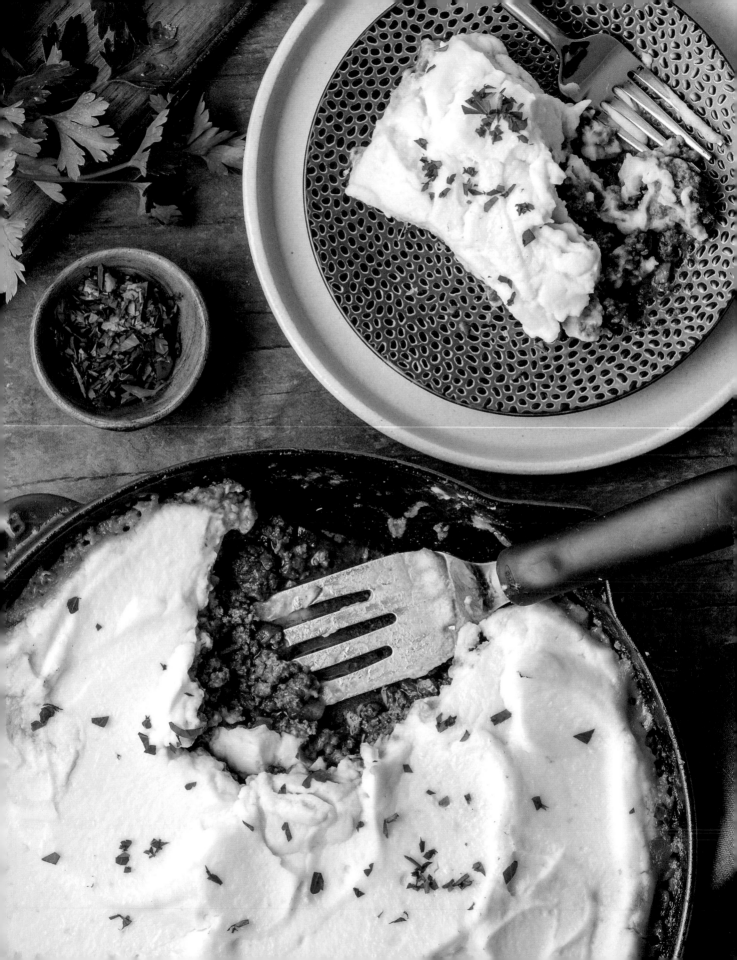

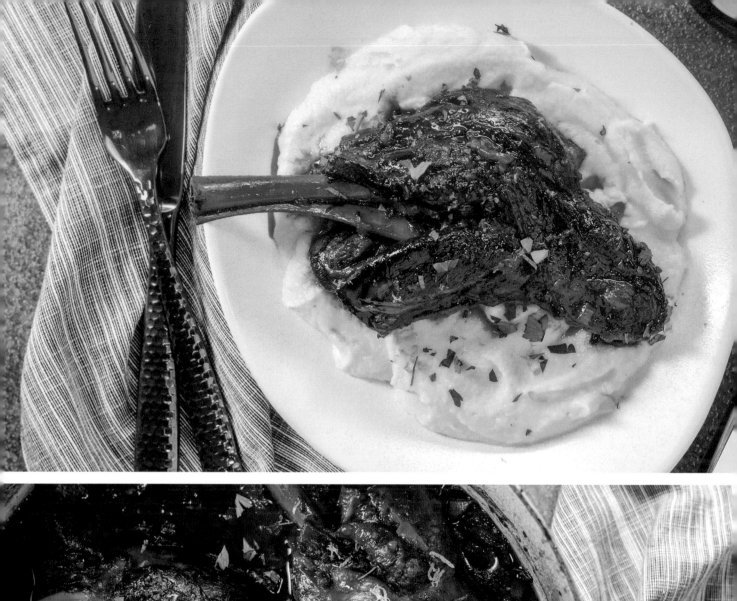
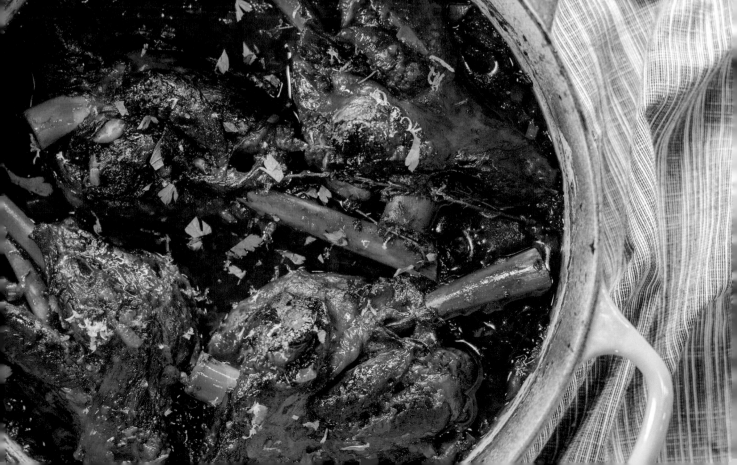

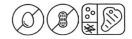

PREP TIME: **15 MINUTES** • COOKING TIME: **3 HOURS** • MAKES: **5 SERVINGS**

BRAISED LAMB SHANKS
WITH CHEESY CAULIFLOWER MASH

This is low and slow comfort food done right. I love to braise tough pieces of meat for 3 hours to the point where the meat gets so tender, it just falls off the bone. Of course, you need something to sop all of those yummy juices, and my cheesy cauliflower mash will play that role perfectly.

 Tip

You can make this recipe using a slow cooker set for 8 hours. I find that an electric pressure cooker is not quite big enough to hold this many lamb shanks, but, if you want to cook fewer shanks, pressure cook on high for 1 hour.

FOR THE LAMB SHANKS:

- 5 lamb shanks
- 1 red onion, chopped
- 2 stalks celery, chopped
- 2 teaspoons fresh thyme, chopped
- 2 teaspoons fresh rosemary, chopped
- 3 cloves garlic, minced
- 3 tablespoons tomato paste
- ½ cup red wine
- 28-ounce can crushed tomatoes
- 1 bay leaf
- 1 quart of beef stock or water
- Kosher salt and fresh pepper
- Olive or avocado oil

FOR THE CAULIFLOWER MASH:

- See recipe on page 239

Make the lamb shanks. Season the lamb shanks with a generous pinch of salt and pepper all around and allow to sit at room temperature for 20 minutes before cooking. Preheat oven to 325°F and preheat a large Dutch oven over medium-high heat with 2 tablespoons of oil. Working in two batches, add the shanks to the pot and brown well on all sides. This will take about 8 minutes. Repeat with second batch and move lamb shanks aside.

Turn the heat down to medium and add the onions, celery, thyme, rosemary, ½ teaspoon salt, and a few cracks of pepper. Cook for 10 minutes and then add the garlic and cook until the veggies are very soft. Add the tomato paste and cook for two minutes, then add the wine. Cook for 3 minutes, or until most of the wine has evaporated, and then add the lamb shanks back to the pot, along with the tomatoes and enough stock/water to come just above halfway of the lamb shanks. Add another ½ teaspoon of salt, the bay leaf, and a few cracks of pepper, and move everything around so the cooking liquid is mixed. Place a lid on the pot and cook in the oven for 1½ hours. Next, flip the lamb shanks, and cook another 1½ hours. Remove from oven and allow to rest with the lid on for 20 minutes before serving. You know the lamb is ready when it pulls apart easily with a fork.

Make the cauliflower mash while the lamb shanks are cooking. Follow the instructions on page 239.

Serve the lamb shanks with the cauliflower mash and reserved cooking liquid and enjoy!

STORAGE AND REHEATING: Everything will keep in the fridge for five days or can be frozen for two to three months. Reheat in a 350°F oven for 10–15 minutes or cover container with wet paper towel and gently reheat in microwave.

MACROS

per lamb shank (makes 5):
449 calories
7.7 grams of net carbs
11.1 grams of total carbs
23.4 grams of fat
44 grams of protein
3.2 grams of fiber

MACROS

per serving of cauliflower mash (makes 5):
91 calories
4.5 grams of net carbs
8 grams of net carbs
4.4 grams of fat
5.2 grams of protein
4.2 grams of fiber

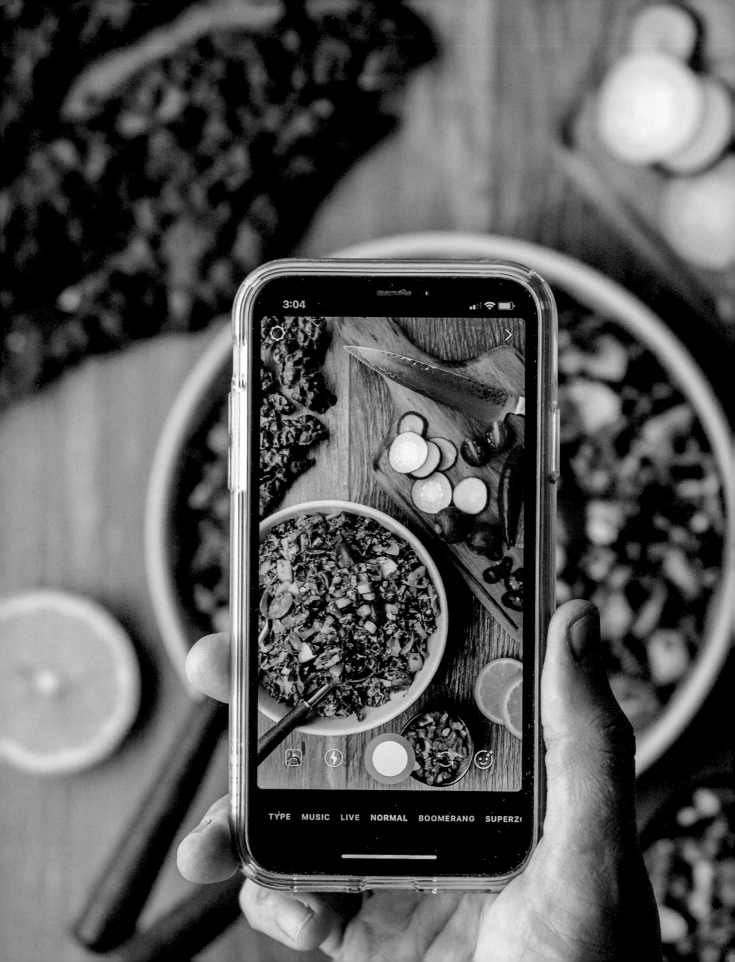

MAMA SAYS: EAT YOUR VEGGIES!

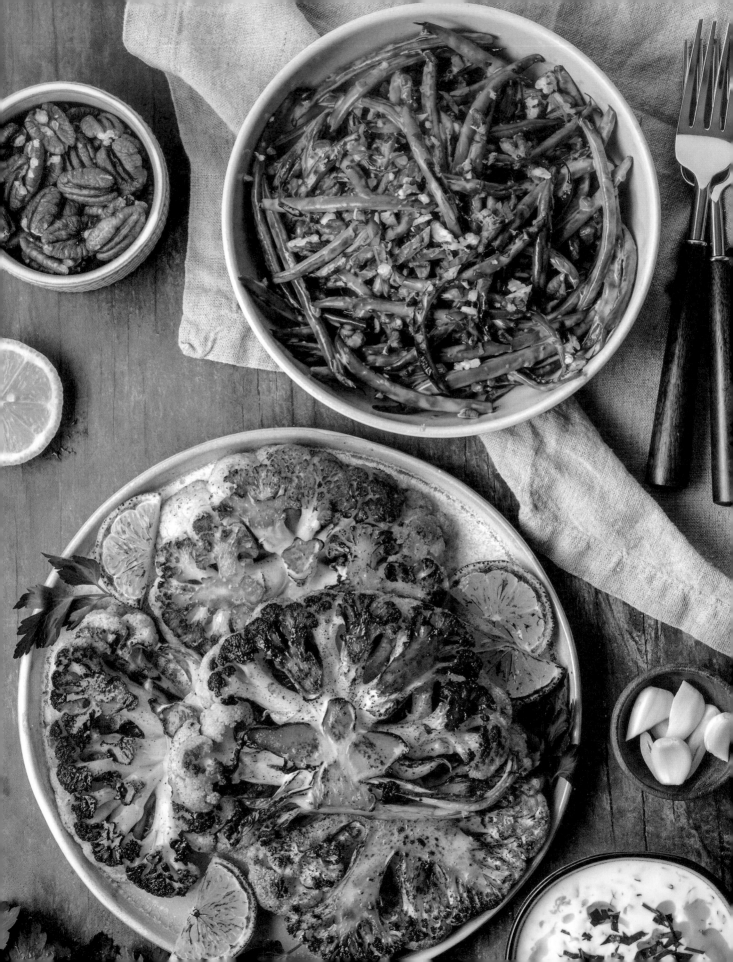

PREP TIME: **10 MINUTES** • COOKING TIME: **30 MINUTES** • MAKES: **5 SERVINGS**

CRUSTY CAULIFLOWER STEAKS
WITH INSANE GREEN BEANS

If you have been waiting for a vegetarian keto meal prep recipe, this one is for you. Meaty spice-crusted cauliflower steaks with a tangy yogurt dipping sauce and quite possibly the tastiest green beans you will ever put in your mouth! Don't be scared by the amount of ingredients for the green beans; they are worth it.

Tip | To make this recipe vegan, use almond or cashew yogurt and vegan mayo.

FOR THE CAULIFLOWER:

- 2 large heads of cauliflower
- 1 teaspoon smoked paprika
- 1 teaspoon ancho chili power
- 1 teaspoon cumin
- ½ teaspoon dried thyme
- Avocado oil
- Kosher salt and fresh pepper

FOR THE YOGURT SAUCE:

- ¾ cup full-fat, Greek-style yogurt
- Zest and juice of ½ lemon
- 2 teaspoons freshly chopped dill
- 1 teaspoon extra virgin olive oil
- ¼ teaspoon kosher salt
- Couple cracks of fresh black pepper

FOR THE GREEN BEANS:

- ⅓ cup full-fat, sugar-free mayonnaise
- 1½ tablespoons lemon juice
- tamari soy sauce
- toasted sesame oil
- 1 teaspoon sambal oelek or sriracha sauce
- 1 teaspoon stone-ground or Dijon mustard
- 1 pound green beans or haricot vert
- ¼ cup red onion, minced
- 2 cloves garlic, minced
- ¼ cup pecans, chopped
- Kosher salt and fresh pepper
- Avocado oil

For the cauliflower steak, preheat oven to 450°F. Cut the ends off both heads of cauliflower—the parts that don't have the root attached. Cut the cauliflower into ¾-inch thick steaks, going from top to bottom and through the stem. You should be able to get six steaks, although the recipe calls for five.

Make the steak spice rub by combining the smoked paprika, ancho chili powder, cumin, and thyme in a small bowl. Mix well. Drizzle a shot of oil on both sides of the steaks. Season with a generous pinch of salt and spice rub on both sides. Place the steaks on a sheet tray and bake for 15 minutes. Remove from oven and set aside. Cauliflower steaks can sit at room temperature for a while after they have been baked.

Make the yogurt sauce by combining everything in a bowl and mixing well. Check for seasoning, you want the flavor to be lemony. Set aside.

Make the dressing for the green beans by adding the mayo to a bowl along with the lemon juice, 1½ teaspoons tamari, ½ teaspoon sesame oil, the sambal, mustard, ¼ teaspoon salt, and a couple cracks of pepper. Mix well and check for seasoning as you may want more spice or lemon juice. Set aside.

For the green beans, preheat a large non-stick pan just below high heat for 2 minutes with 2 teaspoons of oil. Add the green beans and cook for 7–8 minutes, until blistered on the outside, but still crunchy. Add the onions, garlic, pecans and cook for 1 minute. Turn the heat down to medium and add 1½ tablespoons of tamari, ½ teaspoon of sesame oil, and a ¼ teaspoon of salt to the pan and cook for 30 seconds so the beans can steam. Remove from heat and transfer to a large bowl. Once the beans have cooled slightly, add enough dressing to coat.

To finish cooking the steaks, preheat a large cast-iron pan over medium-high heat with 1 tablespoon of oil for 2 minutes. Use a spatula to carefully place 2–3 of the cauliflower steaks in the pan and sear for 2–3 minutes or until the steaks are nicely browned on the first side. Use a spatula to carefully flip the steaks and sear until crusty. Remove from pan and repeat with remaining steaks.

Serve the steaks with the yogurt sauce and green beans and enjoy!

STORAGE AND REHEATING: Everything will keep in the fridge for five days but can't be frozen as it will get very mushy.

MACROS

per cauliflower steak (makes 6):

71 calories
5.1 grams of net carbs
9.4 grams of total carbs
3.3 grams of fat
3.4 grams of protein
4.3 grams of fiber

MACROS

for all the yogurt sauce:

168 calories
6.2 grams of net and total carbs
8.5 grams of fat
17.3 grams of protein
0 fiber

MACROS

per serving of beans (makes 5):

230 calories
4.9 grams of net carbs
8.5 grams of total carbs
21.2 grams of fat
3 grams of protein
4.33 grams of fiber

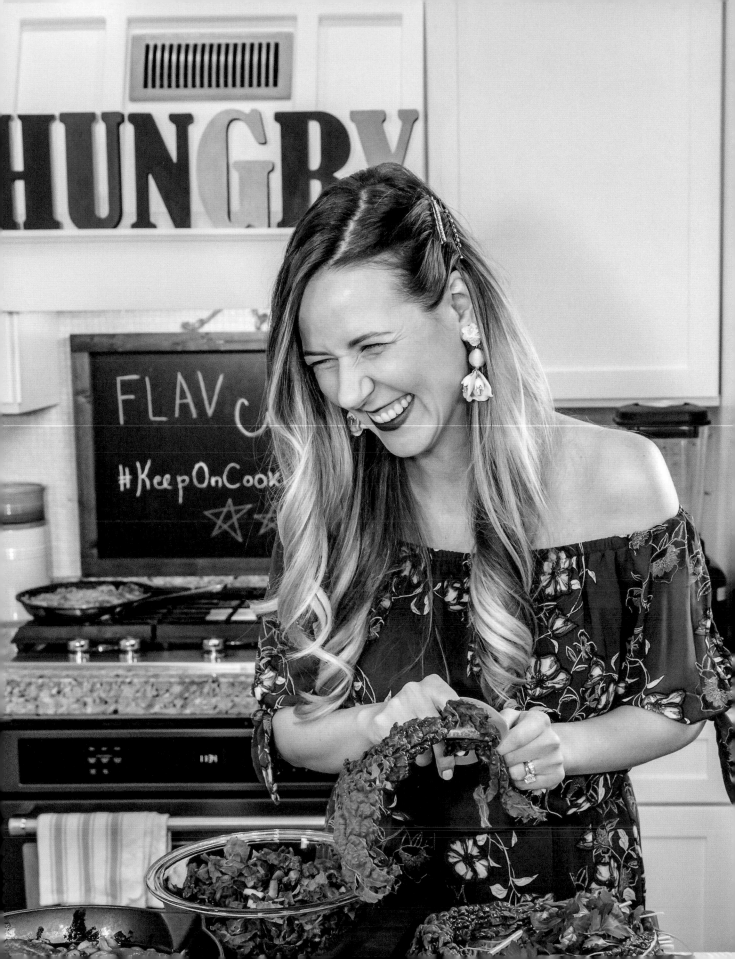

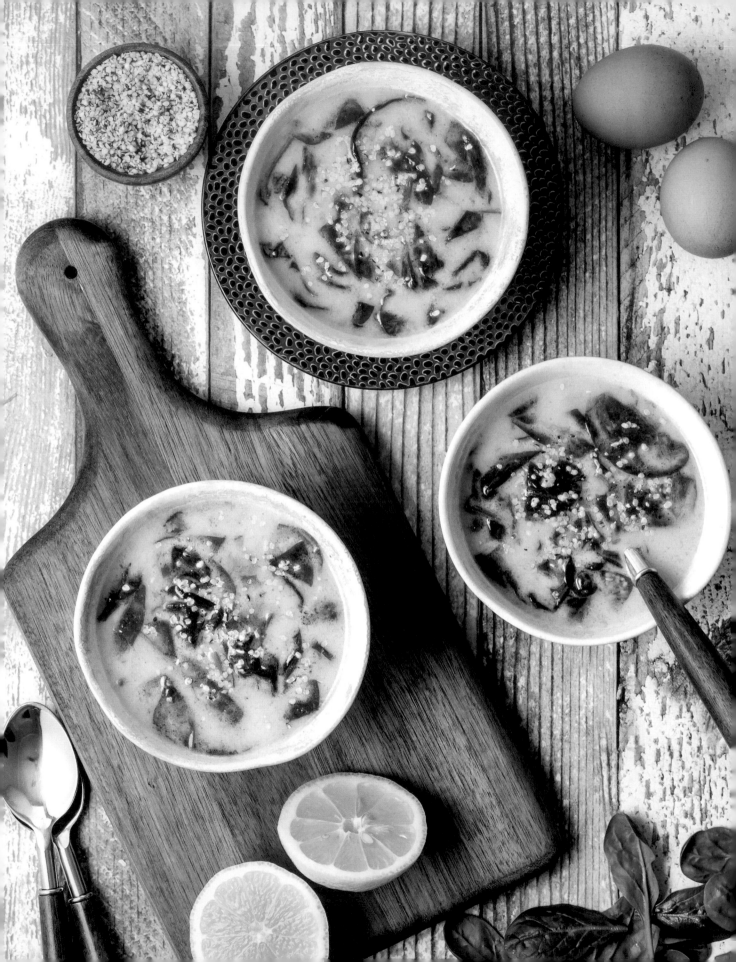

PREP TIME: **5 MINUTES** • COOKING TIME: **25 MINUTES** • MAKES: **5 SERVINGS**

PALEO / WHOLE30

DESSI'S LEMON DROP
SPINACH SOUP

I made this recipe on the FlavCity Instagram story recently and one lady asked me how this can have any flavor since it's only water and lemons! The answer is simple: Zastroika! That's the Bulgarian technique of tempering eggs and lemon to add a rich and creamy flavor to the soup and give it some body. It's such an easy recipe, but, on a cold day, it's exactly what you need.

To watch the video tutorial for this recipe, search "FlavCity fall soups" on YouTube.

INGREDIENTS:

- 2 quarts water
- 12 ounces of baby spinach
- ½ cup shelled hemp hearts
- 2 eggs
- Juice of 1 lemon
- Kosher salt and fresh pepper
- Extra virgin olive oil

Fill a pot with 2 quarts of water and bring to a boil. Add the spinach, 1 tablespoon of kosher salt, a few cracks of pepper, and 1½ teaspoons oil. Reduce to a hard simmer for 20 minutes and then add the hemp hearts and cook another 5 minutes. Turn the heat off the pot.

In a small bowl, whisk the eggs very well, then add the lemon juice. Pass the mixture through a strainer and into a medium-sized bowl. Use a ladle to add a little of the hot soup to the egg mixture while whisking vigorously. This is called "tempering" and will prevent the eggs from scrambling. Keep adding a little bit of the soup while whisking until you've added about 2–3 cups of the hot soup. Make sure the heat is off and add the egg mixture to the pot, mix well, and check for seasoning. The soup will need more salt and perhaps more lemon juice. Season accordingly and enjoy!

STORAGE: Soup will keep in the fridge for three days and can be frozen for three months.

MACROS

per bowl of soup (makes 5):
153 calories
1.2 grams of net carbs
3.1 grams of total carbs
11.8 grams of fat
9.5 grams of protein
1.9 grams of fiber

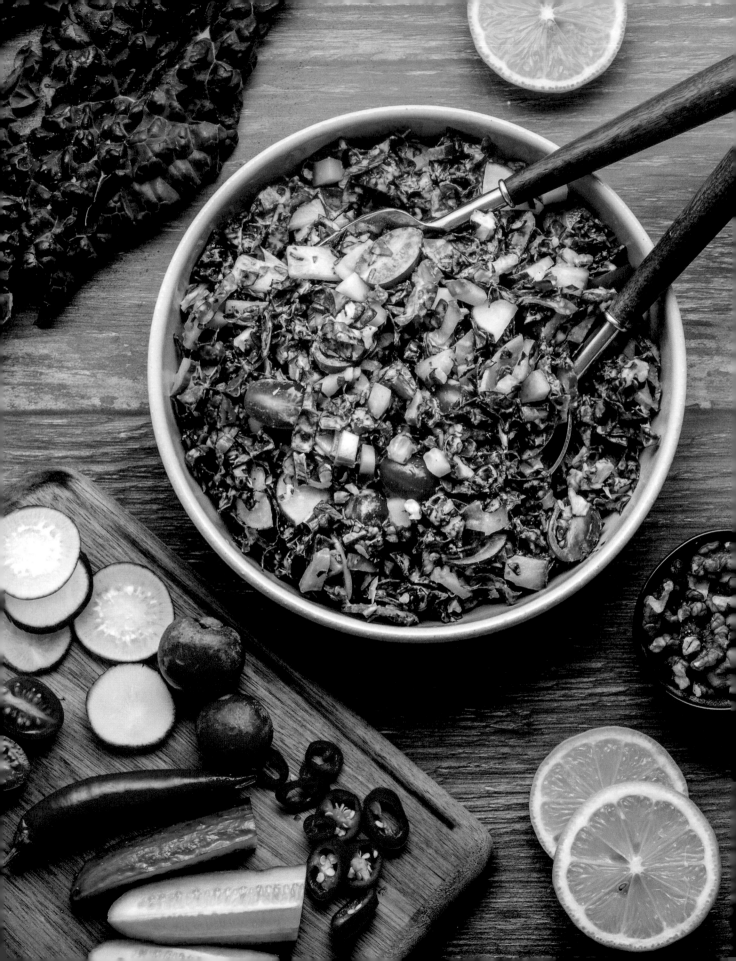

PREP TIME: **10 MINUTES** • COOKING TIME: **1 MINUTE** • MAKES: **1 BIG SALAD**

PALEO

MY FAVORITE LUNCH SALAD

If you follow me on the FlavCity Instagram stories, you will see me eat this lunch salad almost every day during the work week. I call it a garbage salad, because almost any veggies from the fridge will do. I also eat it out of my "dog bowl," a large stainless-steel bowl that I often scrape the bottom of with my fork. It drives Dessi crazy!

 Tip

Look for lacinato kale, also known as dinosaur or black kale. It is softer than curly kale and much more pleasant to eat.

FOR THE SALAD:

- ½ bunch of black (lacinato) kale
- 2–3 radishes, finely sliced
- ¼ cup cherry tomatoes, halved
- ¼ cup seedless cucumber, cubed
- ¼ cup red peppers, diced
- 2 tablespoons toasted walnuts, chopped
- Pinch of salt and pepper

FOR THE DRESSING:

- 2 tablespoons tahini
- 1–2 drops of liquid stevia
- 1 teaspoon stone-ground or Dijon mustard
- 1 clove garlic, finely grated
- 1–2 tablespoons fresh lemon juice
- ¼ teaspoon of salt and couple cracks of pepper
- ¼ cup cold water

Remove the stems from the kale and finely chop the leaves and add to a large bowl along with the remaining salad ingredients. Remember to always add a pinch of salt and pepper to salads. Those veggies are bland and need some love.

For the dressing, add everything but the water to a small bowl. Whisk well and add the water. You may need a touch more water to make the dressing pourable. Check for seasoning as you may want more lemon juice or salt. Toss the salad with the dressing and enjoy!

I often top this salad with a spice-crusted chicken thigh. You can choose any recipe from this book for this purpose. You can't go wrong. Also keep in mind kale is hearty and won't wilt like spinach, so you can dress this salad ahead of time and wait one hour before eating.

MACROS

for one salad:
369 calories
16.1 grams of net carbs
23.5 grams of total carbs
26.5 grams of fat
12 grams of protein
7 grams of fiber

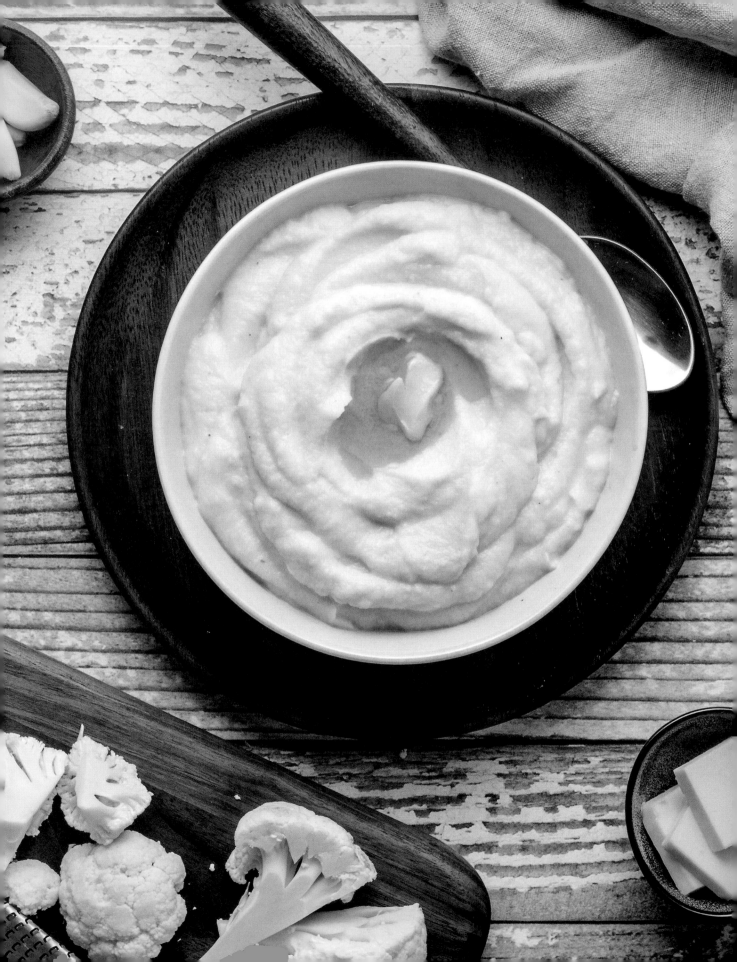

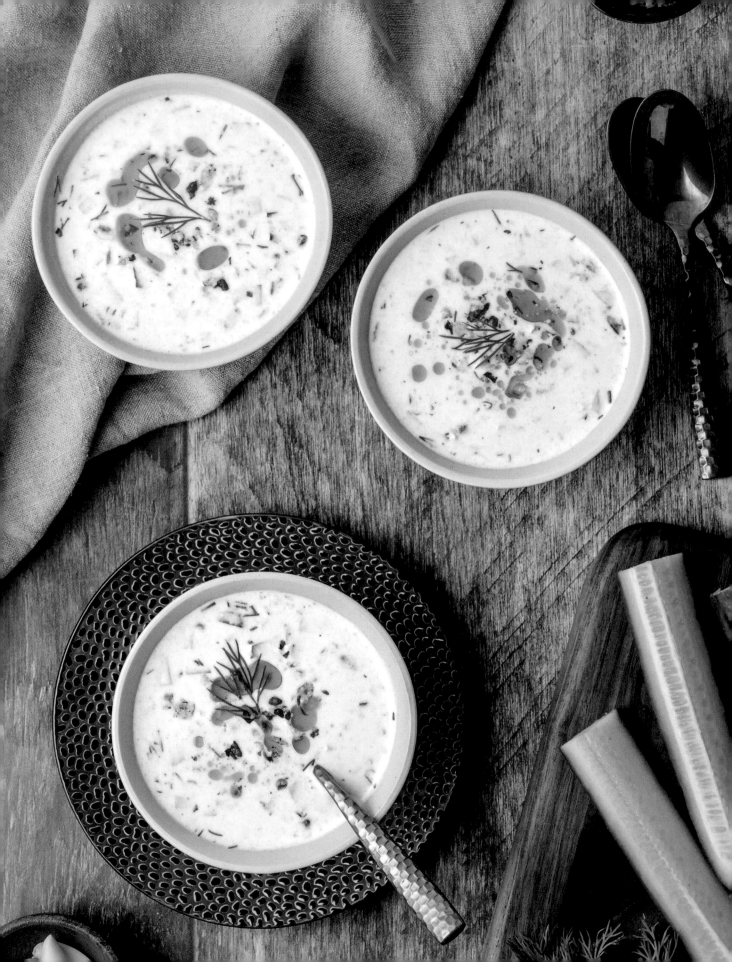

PREP TIME: **5 MINUTES** • COOKING TIME: **1 MINUTE** • MAKES: **2 SERVINGS**

BULGARIAN COLD YOGURT SOUP

This soup literally saved my life on a scorching hot summer vacation in Bulgaria with Dessi. It's exactly what you need on a hot summer day when the last thing you want to do is cook. Drink it cold and, if you're feeling naughty, have it with a piece of banitsa (a Bulgarian filo dough pastry filled with cheese and eggs)!

 To watch the video tutorial for this recipe, search "FlavCity tarator" on YouTube.

- 1 cup full-fat, Greek-style yogurt
- 1 cup cold water
- 1 tablespoon good extra virgin olive oil
- 1 clove garlic, finely grated
- ½ a large seedless cucumber, minced
- ½ cup toasted walnuts, finely chopped
- 2 tablespoons fresh dill, chopped
- 1–1½ teaspoons kosher salt

In a large bowl, add the yogurt, water, and olive oil, and mix well. Add the rest of the ingredients, mix well, and check for seasoning. You may need more salt or possibly more water if the soup is too thick. Place in fridge for up to 4 hours before serving cold.

MACROS

for entire recipe:
702 calories
14.89 grams of net carbs
20 grams of total carbs
58.6 grams of fat
32 grams of protein
5 grams of fiber

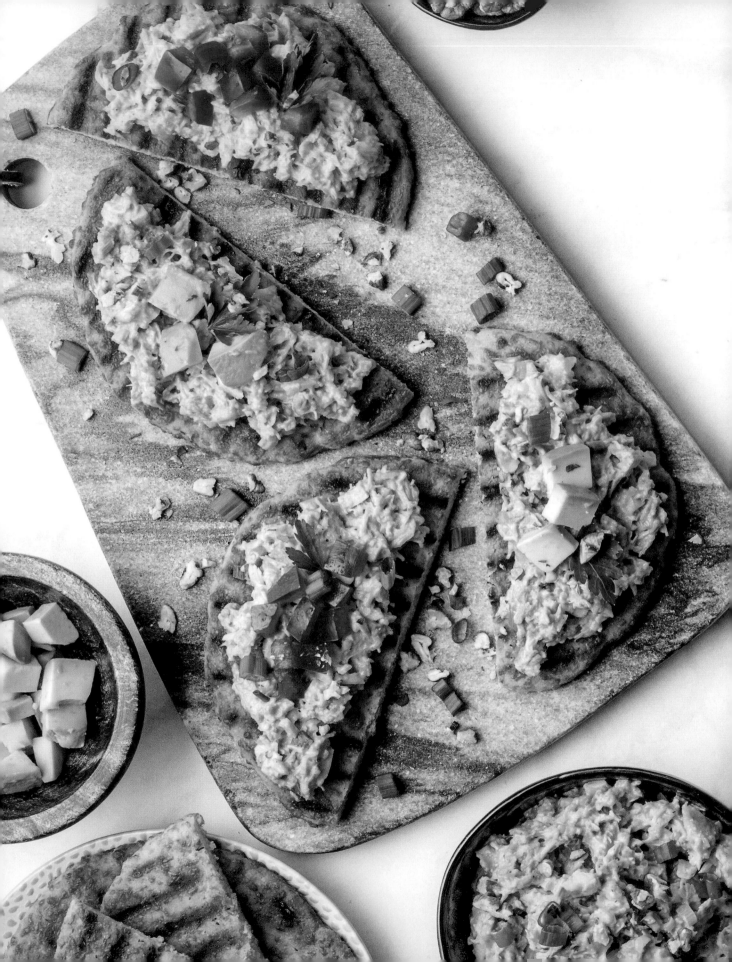

THANK YOU

Big thanks to the FlavCity fans for your support! I truly think of you as family members, and I'm so fortunate to have an amazing community of foodie friends to work with on a daily basis. Thanks for helping us choose the title of this book and for all of the amazing quotes on each recipe—I didn't just make them up!

Thank you to our friends who helped make this book possible. We're not some big production company here folks—it's just Dessi and me. Our good friend Art, who is extremely talented with the camera, helped with many of the food shots in this book and single-handedly did the amazing cover photo for this book! My friend Paul proofread the book, so all of us should be thankful for that, considering I have the grammar skills of a twelve-year-old. Thanks to Rio Chavez for taking the lifestyle photos of Dessi and me. Thanks to Mango Publishing and Brenda for being a joy to work with. We said, "No thanks," twice in the past when book deals came our way, but you guys made it so easy to say "Yes."

ALLERGEN INDEX

Recipe	Page				🚫	WHOLE30	PALEO
WAKEY WAKEY, EGGS AND BAKEY!							
Spinach and Feta Muffins with Butter Coffee	19	✓					
Dessi's Everything Bagels	21			✓			✓
Shakshuka with Feta and Mint	23			✓			
Coffee Shop Egg Bites	25	✓		✓			
Sausage and Veggie Frittata with Ayran	27	✓		✓			
Mini Meatball Breakfast Hash	29	✓		✓	✓	✓	✓
Breakfast Sandwich and Coconut Chia Seed Pudding	31	✓					
Mocha Butter Coffee	35		✓	✓			
Chocolate Chia Seed Pudding	37		✓	✓	✓		✓
WINNER, WINNER, CHICKEN DINNER!							
Moroccan Chicken Stew with Golden Cauliflower Rice	41	✓	✓	✓		✓	✓
Butter-Basted Chicken with Creamed Spinach	43	✓	✓		✓		
Chicken Saltimbocca with Garlicky Roasted Mash	47	✓	✓				
My Best Curry Chicken Salad	49			✓			✓
Creamy Mushroom Chicken and Veggie Mash	53	✓	✓		✓		
Alabama White BBQ Chicken with Black Beans	55	✓		✓	✓		
Roasted Veggie Salad with Fennel-Spiced Chicken Thighs	59	✓		✓		✓	✓
Roasted Chicken Salad with Cloud Bread	61	✓					
One-Pan Coconut Curry Chicken with Veggie Rice	63	✓	✓	✓	✓	✓	✓
Crispy Chicken Thighs with Red Cabbage Crunch Slaw	65	✓	✓	✓		✓	✓
Chicken Fried Cauliflower Rice	69	✓		✓	✓		
Pressure Cooker Chicken Cacciatore with Cauliflower	71	✓	✓	✓	✓		✓

Recipe	Page					WHOLE30	PALEO
PASTA LA VISTA, BABY!							
Gnocchi with Pesto Sauce and Crispy Prosciutto	75	✓					
Greek Chicken with Spaghetti Squash Primavera	77	✓	✓	✓		✓	✓
Asian Salmon Cakes and Noodle Stir-Fry	81	✓	✓	✓			
Ramen Noodle Soup with Pork and Mushroom Wraps	83	✓		✓			
Pesto Pasta with Spice-Crusted Chicken	87	✓	✓				
Fettuccine Bolognese with Arugula Salad	89	✓	✓		✓		
Spaghetti Squash Pesto with Shrimp	93	✓	✓				
Beef Lettuce Wraps with Sesame Noodle Salad	95	✓	✓	✓			
Sesame Chicken and Veggie Stir-Fry	99	✓	✓	✓	✓		
BEEF—RAISING THE STEAKS							
Beef Chili and Cheddar Biscuits	105	✓					
Coffee-Rubbed Skirt Steak with Salsa Verde	109		✓	✓	✓		✓
Nonna's Meatballs and Sauce	111						
Cheesy Stuffed Meatloaf with Broccolini and Eggplant	113	✓			✓		
Beef Kefta with Veggie Pilaf and Yogurt Sauce	117	✓	✓				
Beefy Stuffed Peppers with Tomato Sauce	119	✓	✓				
I SEAFOOD AND I EAT IT							
Citrus-Glazed Salmon with Roasted Cauliflower Salad	125	✓		✓	✓		
Shrimp Burgers with Jicama Fries and Secret Sauce	129	✓		✓			✓
Crusty Shrimp with Roasted Cauliflower Curry	133	✓	✓	✓		✓	✓
Crispy Skin Salmon with Blistered Snow Peas and Rice Pilaf	135	✓	✓	✓	✓		
Green Curry Shrimp with Cauliflower Rice	139	✓	✓	✓	✓	✓	✓
Pan-Seared Salmon with Wilted Kale and Mushrooms	141	✓	✓	✓	✓	✓	✓
Crispy Coconut Shrimp with Chili Dipping Sauce	145			✓	✓	✓	✓
Epic Salmon Burgers and BBQ Kale Chips	147	✓		✓			✓
Summertime Salmon Poke	151			✓			

Recipe	Page					WHOLE30	PALEO
THE SACRIFICIAL LAMB							
Lamb Kebabs with Tahini Sauce and Pita Bread	217	✓					
Spiced Lamb Shoulder Chops with Green Bean Salad	219	✓	✓		✓		
Rebellious Shepherd's Pie and Veggies	223	✓	✓		✓		
Braised Lamb Shanks with Cheesy Cauliflower Mash	227	✓	✓		✓		
MAMA SAYS: EAT YOUR VEGGIES!							
Crusty Cauliflower Steaks with Insane Green Beans	231	✓					
Dessi's Lemon Drop Spinach Soup	235			✓	✓	✓	✓
My Favorite Lunch Salad	237		✓	✓			✓
Buttery Mashed Cauliflower	239		✓		✓		
Bulgarian Cold Yogurt Soup	241		✓				

INDEX

E

F

G

J

K

T

V

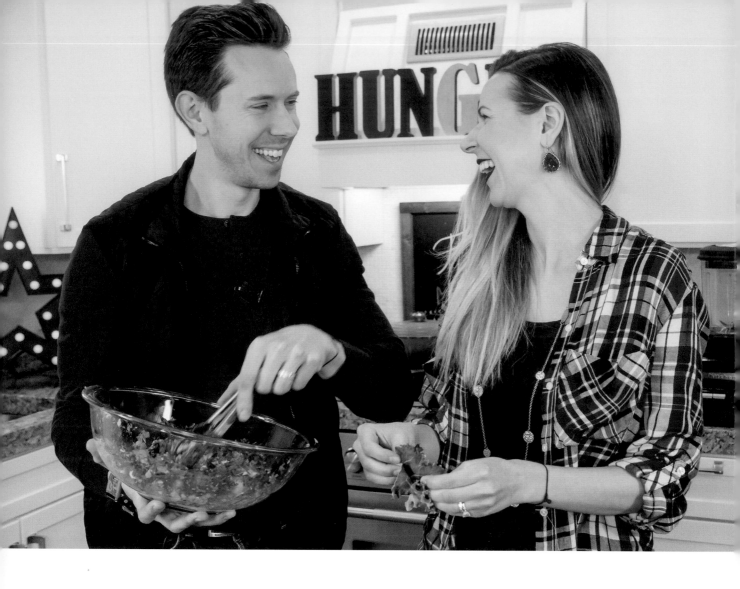

ABOUT THE AUTHORS

Bobby and Dessi have been married for nine years and live on the north side of Chicago in a two-bedroom condo that now looks like a production studio. Dessi is a talented artist. You can see all of her art work at www.dessiart.com.

When not filming videos or creating recipes, you can find Bobby at the gym or shopping at Whole Foods, Trader Joe's, or Costco on a daily basis.

To see more recipes and videos, make sure to subscribe to the FlavCity YouTube channel and follow FlavCity on Instagram, Facebook, and at www.flavcity.com.